Praise from Doctors for
RUSSELL BRANJORD & SPIKE DIET X

"To be honest I have always believed in the "staggered calories"
approach -- the fact of the matter is this: The body fights to
preserve a constant, stable state known as homeostasis. The body
does not like change, it does not want to change --and it will
adjust and up- and down- regulate its internal metabolic milieu
and handling of nutrients and calories to prevent that change. So
varying daily calories has always made intuitive sense to me. But
I'd never seen it laid out in writing in a program until I came
across Spike Diet. I think it has the potential to be the next big
thing.

This is the first "diet" that makes sense to me from a physiology
standpoint -- the body hates to change, rather, it always strives to
maintain homeostasis. Only the truly genetically blessed can
avoid this physiologic near-certainty -- for the rest of us, it doesn't
matter what diet we follow, if it stays the same, the body will
adjust and adapt and alter its internal biochemical and hormonal
milieu, and that diet will stop working, period! I have always
known this from my medical knowledge, and I have personally
experienced it many times. Yet I have never seen a diet that
acknowledges this and works around it, until now!"

-Dr. Andrew Gomes, MD

continued...

"I've known Russ for several years, and I've always admired his passion for helping people lose weight and improve their health. If you are struggling with your weight, it's important that you know he was once just like you. Russ has taken his journey of losing over 100 pounds, and combined this with his research into the most effective methods for losing weight to create his Spike Diet and Spike84 program. Between his personal experience, the results he's seen helping others lose weight, and the research to support his program, you have a very smart strategy that anyone should be able to follow and see great success in losing weight.

By making the decision to take back control of his health and by losing over 100 pounds, I truly believe that Russ has saved his own life! At the very minimum, he has saved himself from a life of misery and unnecessary medical problems. Once you make the decision to take back control of your health, he can help you do the same by following the Spike Diet plan."

-Dr. John W. Larson, DC, DCBCN
Board Certified in Clinical Nutrition
Weight Loss Success® Expert

"Russell has developed and novel weight and body fat reduction system that allows you to maximally use your metabolism achieve results. After investigating more myself, I found out Mr. Branjord was just like myself. He struggled with weight most of his life until he decided to take control of it. He has amazingly transformed his body by losing over 100 pounds and the body of many others using his "novel" nutrition plan. What makes this so extraordinary is that he understands that the human body is a smart organism. The body wants to reach a steady state and that is why people "plateau" when they diet. He took that fact and worked the metabolism to re-feed it (Spike), so that the body feels fed and continually guessing. The body continues to burn fat as the nutrition plan satisfies the body's psychological and hormonal needs to continue weight and fat reduction. The "Spike" manipulates our use of the hormones Leptin and Ghrelin to keep our body losing weight, torching fat, and stoking our metabolism for success.

I contacted Russell to learn more about his nutrition concept and the rest is history. I had to align myself with such an innovative and motivating individual looking to help others with obesity just as I have pledged to do myself.

This is why as a medical professional, I unequivocally endorse Russell Branjord and Spike Diet as an effective weight loss and weight maintenance plan. I share his plan with my friends and patients as the best way to lose weight avoid common diet plateaus and keep your metabolism firing."

-Christopher L.P. Balgobin, MD

Dr. Balgobin's weight-loss success story was featured on local newspapers, NY Times, Network TV Stations and also appeared with Dr. Sanjay Gupta on CNN

"ASK AND IT WILL BE GIVEN TO YOU; SEEK AND YOU WILL FIND; KNOCK AND THE DOOR WILL BE OPENED TO YOU."
-MATTHEW 7:7

SPIKE DIET X

OBESE TO SIX-PACK
HOW I ESCAPED "DIET HELL"

A LIFESTYLE FITNESS PLAN FOR THOSE WHO LOVE TO EAT

WRITTEN BY
RUSSELL BRANJORD

FORWARD BY
CHRISTOPHER L.P. BALGOBIN, MD

ISBN-10: 1542329434
ISBN-13: 978-1542329439

Find more about Living the Spike Life at: www.SpikeGuy.com
Facebook - www.facebook.com/spikediet

MEDICAL DISCLAIMER

The information contained herein is not intended to be a substitute for
professional medical advice, diagnosis or treatment in any manner. Always seek
the advice of your physician or other qualified health provider with any questions
you may have regarding any medical condition.

Always consult a qualified medical professional before beginning any nutritional
program or exercise program. The exercise suggestions are not intended to
substitute for proper medical advice. The author and contributors in this book
assume no responsibility for injuries suffered while practicing any exercise
program. If you have any chronic or recurring conditions such as high blood
pressure, neck or back pain, arthritis, heart disease etc., please seek your
physician's advice before starting any new exercise program.

Other books by Russell Branjord

Spike Diet: A Lifestyle Guide to Indulgent Eating and Burning Fat
Book by Russell Branjord
Originally published: October 7, 2009
Author: Russell Branjord

Living the Spike Life: Eat what you love and lose weight!
Kindle Book
Publication Date: June 3, 2014
ASIN: B00KRO8USI

Coming in 2018
Live and Let Diets Die:

All endorsements and testimonials in this book were given freely without
compensation.

This book is written for those who like me, have struggled for years with trying to lose weight, and also like me, they refuse to give up their dream.

My heart is with you because I know what it feels like to be on the other side of the diet book. Starting a new plan typically begins with a favorable mix of hope and excitement that over time morphs into an unfavorable mix of shame and guilt.

Not on my watch!

While this book contains every bit of knowledge, every trick, and every tool I used to lose 130 pounds over the last 13-years, life happens.
The path no matter how amazing will sometimes become a bit rough.
If you are struggling, please reach out to me either on the Spike Diet Facebook page or email. The one thing you cannot do, is give up.

When you buy my book you join the Spike Community and you'll receive the support of the community and from me personally.

How to Connect with Me

- facebook.com/spikediet
- spikediet@gmail.com
- spikeguy.com

HE GIVES STRENGTH TO THE WEARY AND
INCREASES THE POWER OF THE WEAK.

ISAIAH 40:29

THIS BOOK IS DEDICATED TO THOSE WHO HAVE BEEN MADE TO FEEL
THEY ARE NOT WORTHY OF KINDNESS.
YOU ARE WORTHY OF FAR MORE! YOU ARE WORTHY OF LOVE

Thank you God, for eventually answering my childhood prayer to be skinny and be able eat whatever I wanted on birthdays and holidays without gaining weight.

Thank you to my wife Nichole for loving me even when I was fat. My children, Katie, Isaac, Elijah and, Samuel for inspiring me to live a life full of passion and wonder.

My mom, for all the love, hugs and words of encouragement on those days I'd come home from school crying from being teased. I'd quickly go from feeling worthless to special again in your arms. Without you, I'm not sure if I could have made it through.

And, On that Note

A special thank you to the bullies in my life for inspiring me to dream the impossible dream of going from obese to six-pack. They taught me that because I was fat, I was "disgusting" and not worthy of kindness.

Without this deep rooted childhood pain, I don't know if I would have had the perseverance to never give-up on my dream, even when it was more of a nightmare.
So, it is with full sincerity that I say "Thank you"

JESUS LOOKED AT THEM AND SAID,
"WITH MAN THIS IS IMPOSSIBLE, BUT WITH
GOD ALL THINGS ARE POSSIBLE."

MATTHEW 19:26

The Bumpy Path to Releasing my Second Book

A lot has happened in the 10 years since Spike Diet was originally released. In 2011 the same publisher approached me about writing a new book. He promised this one would be bigger and better and we'd have real PR and marketing. Of course, I said "yes!"

The plan was to release my new book in October of 2012; all I had to do was write my book and finish by the deadline, they'd take care of everything else.

I couldn't hold back the excitement and I didn't want to hold it back! So despite some worries that this was too good to be true. I went ahead and told everyone; friends, family, colleges, strangers walking by on the street.

By the spring I was done with my book and it was going on to a few months of editing and other behind the scenes stuff. The publisher put the manuscript into some review process and the initial reviews I read were very positive.

Then, as if I couldn't be even more excited, the PR firm sent me my itinerary for a 12 city launch tour! I had my future in my hands, quite literally. My future was going to begin at the Barnes & Noble on 5th Ave in New York and finish several weeks later in Los Angeles. Each city had network TV appearances and signings at their biggest bookstores. At this point, I could hardly sleep and I was counting down the days.

Then, as I'm sure you could have guessed, my future began crashing down. I am thankful it crashed down before I was on the plane.

When summer hit, everything with this cooled down. I stopped getting calls and emails with updates. At first, I thought that we're just at the point where we wait, so I did. Another week and more nothing. So I called the publisher and the phone just rang. I emailed him and days went by with no response. The PR firm called me and asked if I'd been able to get a hold of the publisher because they weren't returning her calls either. I asked if I should be worried and she said, probably not, she'd make some calls to find the scoop for the both of us.

Well, there was no need to find it because the scoop found me. One of the publisher's designers, whom I became friends with during the process, called me to say that he was just laid-off and I need to call the owner asap. I told him that I'd been trying for weeks with no luck. He gave me another number and said I should call as soon as we hang up. So, I immediately called the new secret number and he answered! I could tell that he was surprised it was me. He started by saying he was sorry, then proceeded to tell me that his company was in the process of filing bankruptcy. Everything we'd been working for; the tour, TV appearances and my book, they're finished, he said, and he's sorry but there's nothing he could do. I wanted to be angry with him but I couldn't. I could tell he was in tears as we spoke and I realized that his dream came crashing down with mine. I didn't know what to say, I was heartbroken and on the verge of a panic attack. After the initial shock wore off, a feeling of loss and embarrassment took over. I didn't want to give up yet because I couldn't face it. So I became desperate! Willing to do anything, even sell my soul if it came to it.

I thought if I found a new publisher or new investor quickly we could still follow the current plan and make it all happen!

The dream was still alive!

Then I got a call back from a publisher and he seemed interested. He quickly lost interest when he asked me if I had a signed letter granting the rights of the book back to me. The bankrupt publisher still owned the rights to my book.

Dream now dead again.

I didn't get the legal rights back until the following year and by then it was too late. The momentum and hype were completely dead. I didn't have any options in front of me and I was too hurt to try it all over again.

So honestly, I didn't even care that I got the rights back. I didn't care because quite frankly, I quit!

I gave up on this ridiculous dream! Who did I think I was anyway?

I felt stupid for even hoping that something that amazing would happen to me. It was about time I faced the truth. I was born to live an ordinary life and there's nothing wrong with that.

Now, almost 5 years later I realized the sad irony of the situation. I gave up on this dream as I gave up on my dream to lose weight. I wasn't born to live an ordinary life just as I wasn't born to be fat. I naively chose these lives.

I refuse to quit! No matter how long it takes.

I'm not used being so worried about being made fun of. I totally wimped out. I'm sorry. I used to say that my skin was as thick as the body-fat beneath it. I can thank the bullies for that after years of desensitization. Well, I guess with the weight gone I lost my immunity for a while.

The truth is, I know releasing this book, not professionally edited and without a publisher and their "final touches", I am opening myself up to ridicule for errors. But I also know I can't afford a professional editor or afford more time. If I use that excuse I'd just sit on this book for another 5 years. So be warned, this book will have grammatical mistakes.

I also tend to ramble and I'm pretty sure I rambled a few too many times in this book. Yet, I'm not waiting for another proof-reader so go ahead and call me "The Rambler", its okay.

Yeah, some may snicker and talk behind my back because they think I'm either crazy or an idiot or possibly even a crazy idiot, to believe that my book could actually make a difference. I'm willing to take that risk.

I also know I will once again be able to read my name next to the word "broscience" on message boards. Look don't get me wrong, I love fitness groups and forums. Most of the time they are extremely helpful and motivating. But sometimes the dieting message boards can become a bit brutal! The truth is, when people disagree they tend to get angry, but when they disagree over diets they can get downright nasty. I think we are loyal to our diets like we are to our sports teams. So don't you dare say your team is better than mine! If you've been on them, you know what I'm talking about. Now I'm rambling again.

Anyway, I don't care what the "hangry" people say anymore. I'll happily be someone's "broscience fool" if I'm another's inspiration. The truth is, even if my book only helps one person transform their life, then I can say that any ridicule today and from my childhood was worth it. That was my purpose and what I forgot when I was so focused on 5th Ave New York.

I am very excited to finally hand over the book I wrote for you 5 years-ago.

God Bless,

Russell Branjord

HE WHO OVERCOMES WILL INHERIT THESE THINGS
-REVELATION 21:7

SPIKE DIET X FOREWORD
by Christopher Balgobin, M.D.

Unfortunately, we live in the land of ever increasing obesity and the explosive health care costs associated with such a preventable condition. We, as a nation, spend more money on weight loss supplements and health clubs than ever before. We are land of chronic dieters. We jump from one diet to the next in the hope that this of the right one. The statistics are dismal regarding weight loss and weight management. It is estimated that only 5% of people who have lost 30 pounds or more will maintain that weight loss after 5 years. We are living part of an oxymoron of billion dollar spending on the fitness industry yet ever increasing obesity and diseased states associated with this condition. Obesity has been labeled as "epidemic" and the health care costs associated with this condition has reached astronomical levels. We are becoming a sicker population despite having some of the best healthcare in the world. Insurance premiums have become nearly unaffordable for most people and many go without medical insurance as the healthcare cost burden has become too great.

As a full-time practicing Family Medicine Physician, I am on the front lines of the battle. Not a day goes by when a patient comes in asking for weight loss and dietary advice. But to be honest with you, the vast majority of physicians are not adequately trained in nutrition and weight loss management. We often give false information on how to adequately lose and maintain weight. We tell people all sorts of things such as low fat, low carbohydrate, low calories, exercise more, begin juicing, eat whole wheat, eat gluten free, become a vegetarian, etc. Patients, including health professionals are confused about what really to do to lose and maintain a healthy weight and preserve or improve their health.

I have become an expert in fitness, nutrition and weight loss by my own self-study, my own self-realization journey and living it day to day. For those who may not know, I was an unhealthy, morbidly obese physician. When I started my practice, I tipped the scales at 304 pounds on my 5 foot 6 inch frame body. I was giving advice to people on health and weight management despite having my own setbacks. I felt like a hypocrite. I would see patients with diabetes and high blood pressure and hyperlipidemia and knew that my fate would eventually be the same if I did not act. Enough was enough!

To give you some background, I was an overweight kid most of my life. I was active in sports but I eat too much. Every year I got bigger and bigger.

Even as a child was a chronic dieter. I grew up being a chronic dieter. I tried almost every diet known. Every year I would try to lose weight with success most of the time losing up to 20-30 pounds. The success however never lasted. I became more progressively frustrated as I grew older with my weight. I continued to be more focused on doing well in school and my career path, than on my own health. This misdirection lead me to a weight of 304 pounds and a BMI (body mass index) of 46! I reached the point where I thought obesity was my destiny because of my family history and my numerous previous failure attempts at weight loss. I gave gastric bypass a consideration, but quickly gave that up because I didn't want to alter my internal organs to lose weight. So during the winter of 2006-2007, my wife and I made a pledge together to live a healthier life. We agreed to exercise daily and eat better. This involved cooking more at home and tracking caloric intake. It was actually a cliché' that we made this pledge for a New Year's resolution. My wife wanted to lose 70 pounds and I needed to lose over 100 pounds. We began our journey together on January 1st.

After being strict on calorie consumption and daily exercise, extreme progress was made. I was losing weight fast on my own plan. After 5 months I was down over 80 pounds and after 10 months, I had lost a total of 122 pounds. I was the smallest I have ever been since 7th grade. My wife lost a total of 70+ pounds using a popular weight loss plan. We were new people! It was not easy by any means. I was extremely happy at my success but not happy with the way I looked. After so many months of over-stressing my body and calorie restriction, my body was upset at me. I was now skinny fat. I cardio exercised my body into submission. I was losing my hair and I was weak and fatigued. I scavenged my muscle and destroyed my metabolism. I lost weight but I did it incorrectly. I decided that I needed to look physically healthy despite losing that much weight. I was surprised to find out that after my calorie restriction and extreme dieting/exercising, that my metabolic rate was consistent with what you would find in a 130 pound woman. With a metabolic rate that low, there was no way that I could maintain my weight loss. Therefore, I aligned with a personal trainer to start incorporating weight training and healthier eating. I began reading/studying more about fitness, nutrition, and metabolism. These were things I was never taught in medical school. Next, I set on a new journey for self-improvement in health, body transformation and overall reduction of body fat with less emphasis on overall weight. I became a fan of body building and overall physique development. As my self-awareness continued, I was extremely motivated by my patients and the people around me. My patients began to emulate my behaviors. Some of my patients began to transform their own lives by embarking on their own health journey. I have had patients who've lost from

30 pounds to over 250 pounds that they claim is based from my example and motivation. This is extremely humbling to me to say the least. I have a pair of sisters in my practice that have lost a combined 370 pounds together by natural means. The story of my weight loss travelled. I began getting recognition from local TV news agencies and newspapers as well as national news agencies. I have been honored to have appeared in the NY Times as well as my story featured on a segment on CNN with Sanjay Gupta. I serve as a spokes model for my healthcare system in advertisements. I also have my own Sunday morning medical segment on Fox News in Minneapolis. My life has changed in amazing and unbelievable ways. Opportunities have opened up that were never there before.

My transformation and new found passion for fitness and health has allowed me to be blessed to interact with so many wonderful people. I call it fate, but I believe this is how I became friends with Russell Branjord, creator of the Spike Diet and Spike Life. I heard about Russell from a fitness friend. This friend told me about a concept that Russell Branjord developed that allows people to lose weight but also keep their metabolism going. As I was training for a physique competition to maximally drop body fat, I was unknowingly incorporating some of Russell Branjord's nutrition concepts. Russell has developed and novel weight and body fat reduction system that allows you to maximally use your metabolism achieve results. After investigating more myself, I found out Mr. Branjord was just like myself. He struggled with weight most of his life until he decided to take control of it. He has amazingly transformed his body by losing over 100 pounds and the body of many others using his "novel" nutrition plan. What makes this so extraordinary is that he understands that the human body is a smart organism. The body wants to reach a steady state and that is why people "plateau" when they diet. He took that fact and worked the metabolism to refeed it (Spike), so that the body feels fed and continually guessing. The body continues to burn fat as the nutrition plan satisfies the body's psychological and hormonal needs to continue weight and fat reduction. The "Spike" manipulates our use of the hormones Leptin and Ghrelin to keep our body losing weight, torching fat, and stoking our metabolism for success.

I contacted Russell to learn more about his nutrition concept and the rest is history. I had to align myself with such an innovative and motivating individual looking to help others with obesity just as I have pledged to do myself. This is why as a medical professional, I unequivocally endorse Russell Branjord, the Spike Diet, and the Spike Life as an effective weight loss and weight maintenance plan. I share his plan with my friends and patients as the best way to lose weight avoid common diet plateaus and keep your metabolism firing.

To you and your health,

Christopher L.P. Balgobin, MD
Dr. Balgobin's weight-loss success story was featured on local newspapers, NY Times, Network TV Stations and also appeared with Dr. Sanjay Gupta on CNN

Table of Contents

Part V – Exercise & Spike Life   **Page 138**

Part VI – Supplement Guide   **Page 168**

Part VII – Appendix   **Page 172**

"Spiking has released me from food bondage. I no longer have to starve myself and get nowhere."—Cindy

"As someone who has started and failed at countless diets for 30-plus years, I think I've finally found the solution. The Spike Diet may well save my life."—Lauren

"I've spent my entire life being jealous of the people that can eat whatever they want and lose weight or stay skinny. Now I AM one of those people!"—Corrie

"Spiking has allowed me to take control of my diet, my health and my life. I know that once a week I can eat anything I want, so it's that much easier to follow my nutrition plan for the rest of the week. This isn't a diet. It's a plan for a healthy lifestyle."—Bruce

"Be BOLD! Be DIFFERENT! Be a SPIKER!"—Krystal, Team USA

"After years of dieting I've finally got rid of my food demons. No longer am I obsessively calorie counting, or doing the newest fad diet. I'm just enjoying all of the benefits of spiking. If I want a chocolate bar I'll have one on my spike day. I haven't been hungry once since I started."—Hannah, Northern Ireland

"Spiking allows you to enjoy food and not deprive yourself. It's a healthy lifestyle, not some fad diet. Don't drive yourself crazy worrying about a bad day. Plan it, look forward to it, and enjoy it! Trust me, it's worth it."—Alix

"Spike Life takes the pressure off of hardcore dieting without guilt. Making a diet change like this is one I can stick with! Thanks!"—Andy

"The best part for me, you can eat anything you want (anything—even pizza, ice cream, candy bars...) one day a week, every week!"—Nichole

"You're a hero! Seriously! Spiking is the best 'diet' in the entire world and I'm getting people here in Asia hooked on it too."—Katy

SPIKE LIFE PREFACE
Spike Life is a gift that was given to me so that I could share it with you.

Through many hardships and struggles with my own weight and stress, God has provided me with the guidance and wisdom to develop the greatest lifestyle eating plan I have ever followed. This plan is something I need to share with everyone who is looking to lose weight. I really want to reach those who have struggled with failed diets in the past and maybe feel desperate about their situation. I want to tell you that there is hope. This is a plan for people who love to eat and want to lose weight. Living the Spike Life, I have been able to eat my favorite foods and still lose an amazing amount of weight, but most importantly, I've kept it off.

The Spike Lifestyle has already changed the lives of many. I've been sharing my plan and helping others lose weight since I lost 100 lbs eight years ago. Fitness and nutrition became my passions. What was once my greatest struggle became my greatest strength. My desire for this knowledge, and my joy of helping others, led me to become a Certified Personal Trainer and a Certified Fitness Nutrition Coach. This allowed me to reach even more people who needed help. Then I wrote my first book, *Spike Diet*, and created the extreme 12 Week Fat Burning Program Spike84, which allowed me to get television and radio exposure, bringing the Spike story more into the mainstream. This book, *Spike Life*, is about living the Spike Lifestyle. *Spike Life* is about sharing all of my knowledge of weight loss with you, and then giving you options so that you can customize this philosophy to fit your individual needs. It's not quick-fix diet book so that you can lose twenty pounds in a month. This book is about living a long-term lifestyle that you will love, so that you can get to a healthy weight and maintain it.

Spike Life gives you the tools needed to succeed

- ▶ Quick start guide
- ▶ Daily calorie range chart
- ▶ Sample daily menus
- ▶ Food fullness grades
- ▶ BMI chart
- ▶ Formula to measure and track your body fat
- ▶ Action plans for dealing with cravings
- ▶ Sample exercise plan and home HIIT workout
- ▶ Supplement guide
- ▶ Busting 10 common dieting myths
- ▶ Motivational success stories
- ▶ And more...

After reading Spike Life you will have the knowledge that has made me successful
- ▶ You will be in control over food instead of food controlling you
- ▶ When you are put in difficult food situations you will be able to make the best choices
- ▶ You will learn how to keep your blood sugar stable
- ▶ I will teach you how to efficiently and effectively exercise for only about an hour a week
- ▶ You will know which foods provide us the most benefit to weight loss
- ▶ You will learn the factors that can negatively impact metabolism and weight loss, but more importantly, I will show you how to negate those affects by *spiking metabolism*
- ▶ Spike Life will turn you into a fat-burning machine!

SPIKING IS A LIFESTYLE
This is a long-term lifestyle weight management plan

Spike Life is not a diet. This is not a short-term fix! Spike Life is a manageable lifestyle that has already improved the lives of many. "Spiking" is a unique way to have it all: the body you want, and to indulge in the food you love. It's actually quite simple; six days a week we focus on healthy foods that provide us amazing nutrition and at the same time make us feel fuller so that we won't need to eat as much. Then one day a week, it's anything goes and we are allowed to indulge in whatever we desire. You will see how this philosophy not only gives us a mental break but also manipulates our metabolism so that we are able to lose more weight and keep it off.

There is no "Introductory Phase" in Spike Life

Unlike many diet books, this is the guide to living the Spike Lifestyle. You are not going to start with the standard "Introductory Phase" that is nearly impossible for anyone to stick to. You know the phase where you cut out all carbohydrates, or worse, you're forced to eat only celery sticks and drink lemon juice!

The plan is to continue living the Spike Lifestyle

I'm not going to lie to you and tell you that after you reach your goal weight, you can simply go back to eating the way you used to and expect to keep the weight off. It just doesn't work that way. Our old eating habits made us overweight to begin with and it doesn't change simply because now we are thin. This book is the beginning of a new long-term lifestyle. I want you to become a Spiker for life!

I want spiking to change your life. I want this to be the last weight loss plan you ever need to try. I think some in the diet industry don't care what happens to you after you lose weight. They may feel like their job is done once you hit your goal weight, or worse, once they have your money. They probably expect that if you do lose weight and gain it back that you will come back to them for more short-term help. Often we do; we assume the plan worked because we did lose weight and it was our fault we couldn't maintain it. It's a give and take relationship, you give them money and they take you back. I don't believe success lies in short-term weight loss. Success is losing weight and maintaining your weight loss long-term. This can be done by living the Spike Life.

Spike Life where no food is taboo!

For this to be a happy lifestyle you can't feel deprived. You need to be allowed to eat or drink whatever you want, and I do mean ANYTHING.

You may ask, how can I eat what I want and live a healthy lifestyle?

I have experienced, tested, proved, and also backed with math and science that you can to lose weight with one "bad day" of eating a week.

Like the words out of my favorite book, there's a time to cry and a time to laugh. Just like there's a time for vegetables and there's a time for donuts.

I personally live the Spike Life. I've been doing it now for about 8 years and I have no plans of ever stopping.

Spike Life was a dream of mine that actually came true. When I was young I used to pray that I could eat whatever I want and I'd be thin. Well, it was a miracle. My prayers have been answered. I now eat whatever I want, and I lost over 100 lbs and more importantly, it's stayed off!

Cherish the Journey

I will always cherish the year I lost all of that weight. It was an amazing journey where I really learned the secrets of how my body worked and how it responded to food and exercise. Many of us are in such a hurry to lose weight that we don't take time to enjoy the amazing changes we are making to our body and our mind. This is because dieting typically isn't enjoyable and we just want to be done with it. Dieting can feel like a prison, so of course, we want to just do our time and maybe even get early release for good behavior. With Spike Life I want you to enjoy every pound lost, every Spike Day, and every day of this fabulous journey.

You will not feel deprived living the Spike Life. In fact, it's the most gratifying weight loss plan you will ever try. Every week you will have a Spike Day to look forward to, a day that many Spikers describe as *feeling like Christmas*. You will be able to lose weight, build muscle, feel healthier, look younger, all the while still enjoying all of the foods you love.

There will be struggles and obstacles

Even though spiking is incredible, you may still find yourself struggling at times. Because of my personal experiences, I understand these struggles and I know the obstacles we face when we change from our old habits to a healthy lifestyle. Spike Life helps you succeed by addressing the obstacles your body, and life in general, will throw at you throughout your journey.

Spike Life has an action plan for dealing with each obstacle you may encounter while losing weight:

- ▶ Hunger and cravings
- ▶ Shopping for groceries
- ▶ Eating out
- ▶ Metabolism and hormones
- ▶ "Starvation Mode"
- ▶ Exercise and activity
- ▶ Busy lives
- ▶ Even our *naughty* food cravings

SPIKING WILL CHANGE YOUR LIFE

You are about to join a community of "Spikers" that stretches around the globe. There are Spikers everywhere! People love spiking, and they tell others about it too. The Spiking Community is growing by the minute. The Spiking Community includes: doctors, psychologists, trainers, bodybuilders, athletes, models, actors, TV personalities, and of course amazing moms, dads, teens, families, and everyday heroes that took back control and made a stand to lose weight once and for all.

I've noticed from reading website message boards that Spikers are happy "dieters" that really care about helping others. Many times there are rivalries between followers of different diet plans. They tend to fight constantly on message boards and are sometimes quite mean about it. I remember reading posts on a diet forum from one member pleading with her fellow community members to stop bickering and be nice to each other. The common reply was, "We're cranky and hungry." Spikers are the exact opposite. They are always friendly, happy, and helpful, regardless of what "diet team" the other person is on. I believe this is because Spikers are actually *enjoying* living this lifestyle. Can you imagine dieting and having fun doing it? Spiking gets results! Many Spikers have lost over 100 lbs like I did. Not only are they maintaining the weight loss, but they keep getting leaner and leaner. Some of them have been spiking for years and not only are they successful but they really understand the science and synergy behind the Spike Life. These people I call my "Spike Masters." After you read this book and gain the knowledge you need to take control of your life, I ask that you pay it forward and also help others who need help.

YOU CAN CHANGE THE LIVES OF OTHERS

The world needs to learn about spiking and it needs more Spike Masters to improve the lives of others and reverse the trend of obesity. This is the butterfly affect that I want to create with this book. My struggles made my life miserable, and I eventually regained control over my life and defeated obesity. If it just ended there, I would still be remorseful for the years I lost when I wasn't enjoying my life. I have no remorse now. If I had the choice, I would go through it again and again. My story has helped many reach their goals, but even if I only helped just one person live a happier life. Improving the life of that one person makes the pain of my past worthwhile. I now know there was a reason I struggled, a reason God placed this burden on me. There's also a reason He placed that burden on you. Your story will be the catalyst that will spark the change in another's life. It may be a parent, a child, a sibling, friend, or someone you've never met. Learn this knowledge and share it. Every morning I wake up to messages from people that now have control of their life because of my story and spiking. Believe me, there is no better way to start a day than knowing you are making a difference in the lives of others.

PART I

WELCOME TO THE SPIKE LIFESTYLE

Introduction
My Story

Chapter 1
Introducing the Spike Lifestyle?

Chapter 2
The Current State of Obesity

Chapter 3
Why Dieting Doesn't Work
Dieting as a Quick Fix
Conventional Dieting Myths
Searching for the "Magic Pill"

MY STORY

This is the story of a man that grew up as the fat kid. In school he was bullied for being overweight and he felt helpless about his situation. As an adult his weight became an even worse issue. He was called morbidly obese by his doctors, and at his heaviest, he was over 330 lbs. After the birth of his first son he realized he had to change his life for both himself and his family. He embarked on a weight loss journey that not only improved his life, but now it's improving the lives of others. This is the story of how spiking came to be. This is my story.

MY STORY

My experiences with weight loss will be familiar to many who have struggled with being overweight. I've been on numerous diets; I've lost weight many times, and like most people, I've gained weight back. From my earliest memories I was the "fat kid." If there was ever someone who was destined to be obese, it was me. It's like I was born to be fat. As a kid I didn't know why I was larger than everyone else. I didn't like it but I didn't know what to do about it, or if there even was something I could do about it. I assumed I was just born this way. I didn't want to accept my fate. I wanted to be thin like everyone else. I hoped for a miracle. I starting to pray before going to sleep and I would ask God, "please let me wake up thin." While I never just woke up thin, God did answer my prayer years later when I was ready for it.

At the young age of 13, when I weighed around 230 lbs, I decided enough was enough and I was going to lose weight. Like many in the late 80s I went on a strict regimen of "Sweating to the Oldies," jumping on a mini-trampoline, and a low-fat diet. It worked! I lost over 30 lbs during the summer and when I went back to school in the fall some classmates didn't even recognize me. It was awesome! I vowed to never be overweight again. It just wasn't that easy. Over the next several months and years my weight would fluctuate, up 10 lbs and down 10 lbs, up 20 lbs and down 20 lbs. It's like I had to keep doing more and more, and eat less and less to keep my weight down. I went through long periods of refusing to eat and exercising for several hours a day just to keep myself from gaining weight. I even gave up two of my favorite foods, pizza and ice cream, for a few years. I did whatever I thought was necessary to stick to my vow.

When I was in my early twenties it wasn't as easy for me to dedicate as much time to exercise and I began eating more like a normal young adult would. My weight started slowly going back up. Within a year I was back to my previous heaviest weight of 230 lbs. At first, I didn't just give up. I can't count the number of different diets and exercise plans I attempted and failed. It seemed the more I tried, the more I'd eventually gain.

I was literally out of control; a few years later I had gained over 100 lbs and hit my all-time heaviest weight of 330 lbs. At this point of my life I was married, I had a child, and I was just as depressed as I was obese. I finally did give up and chalked it up to my poor genetics and fate. After all, I was born to be fat.

Then in the summer of 2003 I had a revelation. My son was just over a year old and I did not want him to grow up obese like I did. I didn't want that life for myself and I especially didn't want it for him. I knew that we only have one chance at life and I wanted it to be great! I wanted to be the kind of father that my son would look up to, a father that had the energy and body to play and run around with him. I knew there was a chance that weight was going to be a struggle for him, and I wanted to show him that he wasn't born to be fat. That he could in fact be in amazing shape despite the genetics that I bestowed upon him, because I did it.

With my newfound hope and enthusiasm I began reading everything I could find on nutrition and exercise. I was going to be a master of weight loss and eliminate the uncertainty I used to have when I tried to lose weight in the past. I also began praying as I did as a youth, but not for the miracle of just waking up thin; instead I asked God to help me and give me guidance and the knowledge I needed to finally end my lifelong struggle.

My new plan got off to a great start. I was losing weight fast, three to four pounds a week. Everything was going flawlessly until I was about two months in. For no reason I could think of, I just stopped losing weight. I was tracking and logging every calorie I put in my mouth and I was exercising almost every day— I was perfect. It didn't make any sense, but I was not going to quit. So I just kept going, then another week went with no weight loss, and then another. Now it was really starting to get to me. Besides the fact that the scale wasn't moving, I was getting horrible food cravings, the kind of cravings that can drive you mad. I didn't just want a donut. I was dreaming, and even daydreaming, of eating donuts. I just wanted to hold one so I could feel it, smell it, and guard "my precious." I knew I had a real problem when I was worried I may get banned from my local bakery for drooling on the glass. It got worse when pizza and ice cream began entering my dreams and they would battle with donuts for my affection. I was a wreck, my workouts were suffering, and my job was suffering. I needed to get these foods out of my head but I was not going to quit my diet. Being the perfectionist I was while dieting left me at a strange crossroads. I thought about what I should do for a few days and I came to the conclusion that, despite my diet, I needed to give in to my temptations for just one day. Oscar Wilde once said, "The only way to yield to temptation is to give in to it." Now perhaps he had a different meaning behind the message, but for me this meant I could either live with this temptation and feel deprived the rest of my life, or I could yield to it and end it, with one brilliant day of indulging.

I felt I was still very motivated at the time and this one "bad day" wasn't going to ruin my goals. I did the math and I saw that even if I ate 5,000 calories I would gain one pound at the most. If that one pound of weight gain got my head back on track then it would be more than worth it. I chose to let go of my need for "diet perfection" and I took a day off. That Saturday I ate everything that had been invading my thoughts the past few weeks. It was glorious. I woke up to donuts, I had burgers and onion rings for lunch, I had a huge cookie dough ice cream treat, and I ordered pizza for dinner. Food never tasted so good. Oddly enough, I didn't feel an ounce of guilt for the damage I thought I might be doing. I was simply enjoying the day. The next morning I noticed that I was still satisfied; I could actually think about donuts without going into a psychotic rage. It was no longer "my precious" and just food again. My energy was also much better. My workout later that day was fantastic. That day to indulge did everything that I hoped for, but it actually did more! At the end of the week I weighed myself and I was shocked to see that I lost three pounds! This just blew my mind! I was perfect for three weeks without a single pound lost, and then I ate like there was no tomorrow and I actually lost weight! How was this possible? Did I care? Of course I did it again and again, and over the next several months I lost 100 lbs. This was the beginning of Spike Days. I later found out why they work and learned that I wasn't "cheating"—I was "spiking"! While Spike Days may seem counterintuitive, they actually make perfect sense when you look at the whole picture.

How does eating more help with weight loss? In this book I will show you and you will understand all of the benefits that spiking has on weight loss. After you have learned this knowledge, you will be shocked that Spike Days aren't a part of every diet plan.

Take it One Day at a Time

Spike Life, in a way, is a series of short 6-day diets. You will not be overwhelmed by the enormity of losing 30, 40, 50, or even 100 pounds because all you have to do is focus on today and not worry about tomorrow. You don't have to be concerned about never being allowed to eat your favorite foods, as you won't be more than 6 days away from having a day to eat whatever you want. You also will never have to feel guilty for indulging yourself on a "Spike Day" as it is vital to spiking your metabolism and restoring balance to your mind and body. I can tell you this: after my Spike Day I am ready to go back on my daily calorie diet. I am refreshed and renewed. The Spike Day is like a reset button for your diet. You know how everyone loses weight at the beginning of their diet, before their bodies adapt and weight loss slows down to a screeching halt? Well, every week of Spike Life is the like the first week of a diet for as long as you choose to follow it.

It is important to set daily goals. Daily goals are the steps on the ladder that will help you reach your ultimate goal. For me, daily goals are just staying within my calorie range and then doing something active, whether it was going to the gym, going for a walk, or playing with the kids. We have to get active and we have to move if we want to improve our health. Tell your friends and family your goals. Take that first step and get your support group together. They will marvel at your continued success. There is no fear of failure and no "trying," just doing. You now have the plan, so with faith and determination, you will succeed. I know you can do it, just like I did.

MY PERSONAL MESSAGE TO YOU

My message to you is that even though you may feel you are alone, you're not. Besides myself, there are millions of people who go through days of feeling embarrassed, frustrated, and hopeless because of their weight. I can't count the number of failed diets I have tried in the past, and I'm sure this is also not the first time you have been excited, thinking that this could finally be it—the plan that helps you lose weight forever. The good news is that Spike Life is that plan.

Like you, I've been on many diets where I lost weight initially but, for no apparent reason, I just stopped losing weight. I usually chalked it up to my poor genetics or fate. The last time this happened, though, I would not accept being overweight as my fate. I was frustrated and was determined to understand why my weight loss stopped. I wouldn't be satisfied until I knew exactly why this happened and what I needed to do to finally rid myself of excess weight forever.

I knew it was not a simple solution like "eat less food" or "work out more." I ate far less than many of my thin friends and I exercised more than many of my in-shape friends.

There are so many factors working against us; we're busy, we have sedentary lifestyles, fast food on every corner, the cheapest food is unhealthy food, exercise isn't fun, and ironically, when we attempt to lose weight, even our body works against us. It can be totally overwhelming!

In fact, chances are it is NOT totally your fault you are overweight! This is so important I will say it again: It's NOT your fault! I hate the common stereotypes that all overweight people are lazy and simply lack the willpower to say no. That stereotype is so far from the truth, and so personal, that few other statements cause me as much anger.

The truth is overweight people exercise as often as or even more often than "thin people" do, and most of them are actively trying to improve their health through diet and exercise. If you don't believe me then visit a local gym or look at the billions of dollars thrown at the weight loss industry yearly.

Even though losing weight is difficult, we do have to take control and responsibility for our current weight. I was a glutton. I love to eat food, especially the ones that make us fat, and that love for food definitely was the number one factor in me being morbidly obese. At my heaviest I was over 330 lbs and morbidly obese. My love for fattening foods, and my inability to stay away from them for long periods of time, was also a large reason most diets didn't work for me. Depriving myself of the foods I love drove me into a vicious cycle of feeling sad and deprived, wearing down my willpower until I inevitably gave in. The stress of feeling like a failure perpetuated my poor eating habits until I abandoned yet another diet that wasn't conducive to me…the human being. However, the Spike Lifestyle is my liberation. This plan turned my body into a fat-burning machine while keeping my cravings satisfied and ending my struggle with diets for good! For once I was in control. The short and long-term results created a cycle of another kind: one of weight loss, success, empowerment and positive lifestyle changes.

CHAPTER 1

INTRODUCING THE SPIKE LIFESTYLE

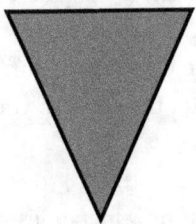

It's time to learn about the Spike Lifestyle. Here you will learn the basic outline of the spiking philosophy, why it works, and why it's different. One of the most important factors to weight management is not allowing food to control you. Spike Life is designed to give you back the control you need to get to and maintain a healthy weight.

Spike Life is true weight loss synergy. It has a plan for all of the physical and mental challenges that dieters face when it comes to losing weight and maintaining it. Spike Life maximizes metabolism and allows you to eat the foods you love while obeying the law of *calories in versus calories out.*

THE BEGINNING OF THE SPIKE LIFESTYLE

The Spike Lifestyle is a weight management plan that is a hybrid of the way we should eat and the way we want to eat. As much as we may want to be healthy 100% of time, the truth is we are not. It's almost impossible to be perfect. This is a fact that is proven by statistics when we are told that over two-thirds of Americans are overweight and quickly growing. Even when we lose weight, the majority of us gain it back. Most of us know what foods are "good" and which foods are "bad," but yet even when we really try to make a change it seems to only last temporarily.

Stay in control by not giving up the foods you love

The problem for me is I love to eat and I love bad food even more. Unfortunately for me this love is true love. I've heard it said that if it's real true love, you can let it go, and if it's meant to be then it will return to you. Well I've let it go dozens of times and my love returned to me over and over again. There's no getting around it, I'm head over heels in love with the wrong kinds of foods. I could never think of food as simply fuel for my body. I get too much joy and pleasure from eating bad foods. I am emotionally connected to bad food for life; when we are apart my heart aches for its prompt return.

My emotional pain was always worse when I'd completely eliminate the foods I love in an attempt to lose weight. It's true that when you can't have something, you want it more than ever. Feeling deprived was almost as frustrating as being overweight. I felt like I had an angel on one shoulder telling me, "You don't need that donut, you're looking great!" And a devil on the other side saying, "Just eat it, one donut won't hurt you." I would do my best to be perfect, but after a while that devil would trick me into eating things I didn't necessarily want to eat, and I'd feel terrible. I really do *not* miss those days.

With the Spike Lifestyle you can have that donut. The difference is *you are in control* and you choose when you do it, not the devil on your shoulder.

There's more to losing weight than eating the right foods

What I didn't know in the past was how metabolism worked, and how diets and even different foods affected my metabolism. I just assumed that if I exercised a lot and ate lots of oatmeal and vegetables, I would lose weight. I thought losing weight was only about eating right and exercising daily. I had no idea that energy or calorie balance was what truly mattered. I also didn't know that my constant dieting and exercise was setting me up for eventual failure.

Spike Life factors in our emotional eating, our physical cravings, our metabolism, our hormones, exercise, and the types of foods that can actually help us lose weight.

I found you can still enjoy the foods you love and lose weight

Do you think you could stick to a weight loss plan, if one day a week you were allowed to literally eat anything you want?

I'm hoping you said yes.

If you said yes, then Spike Life is perfect for you. You can lose weight when once a week you indulged in foods like pizza, ice cream, donuts, cake, or anything else.*Don't believe me?*

I don't blame you for being skeptical. Before I started spiking I would never have believed it. I mean, one day every week I can eat a bunch of donuts and pizza and still lose weight? It sounds almost too good to be true.

Spiking is both good and it's very true. You can and will lose weight if you stick to the calorie goals for you in this book. In fact, I will show you by the numbers how even with a weekly Spike Day you will be in an overall caloric deficit each week. This weekly caloric deficit will result in weight loss.

Spiking makes perfect sense

When you know the facts about calories, metabolism, fat storage, and fat burning, and you also know the emotional aspects of cravings, you will understand why spiking is successful. It's really a no-brainer to come to this conclusion. People "fall off the wagon" and "cheat" on their diets all the time. It happens to all of us and nothing can stop it. It happened to me all of the time until I quit "falling off the wagon" and I chose to "jump off the wagon" on Spike Day instead. When you are in control it is much easier to get right back on the wagon the next day. No hard feelings and absolutely no guilt.

It all began with my first Spike Day eight years ago, when it shocked my body out of a diet plateau and back on the track of weight loss. From that point on I've had a Spike Day every week and I always will, and why not? Instead of that day of indulging making me gain fat, it helped me lose more weight!

SPIKE LIFE IS NOT A DIET BOOK

This is the book you've been waiting for, but it's not a diet book, it's the lifestyle you've been dreaming of. *Spike Life* will forever change the way you think about weight loss and food, and give you the knowledge you need to succeed.

Spike Life is not like the other weight loss books that you may have read, and I am also not like the authors who wrote those books. I created the Spike Lifestyle from my years of personal struggle with obesity. I am not a skinny outsider looking in on the obesity epidemic and proposing my theory on why most Americans are overweight. I'm on the inside. I've battled obesity on the frontlines! I lived and learned the facts about how my body worked and what I needed to do to lose weight once and for all. This knowledge allowed me to finally end my battle and live the life I used to only dream about. Spike Life is the opportunity to be one of the "fit people" and still fulfill your desire to eat the foods that you love oh so much.

Diets are a temporary solution to a permanent problem. If you are looking for a "quick fix" then this isn't the book for you. The goal isn't to lose 20 lbs in 30 days like some books *promise*. My goal is to get you to fall in love with this amazing lifestyle by introducing you to all of the benefits of spiking. I will educate you on how this simple trick, and adopting other clever concepts, will allow you to have it all. I know if you love it you will stick to it. More importantly you will get in amazing shape without ever feeling like you're dieting again. I want Spike Life to become your new lifestyle, not your new diet. What we do on week one, we do on week 100, and on. I tell people all the time that a successful plan isn't losing 20 lbs. A successful plan is losing 20 lbs and keeping it off. According to several major studies and surveys, losing weight short-term isn't difficult, but keeping it off is. 95% of people who lose weight on a diet gain it all back or more within 2 years. While this number is extremely sad, I am one of the rare 5% who has lost weight and kept it off for several years. The reason why I have been successful while so many others haven't is because my diet became my lifestyle. I've never stopped spiking and why would I? I love this lifestyle. I'm a Spiker for life!

WHY IS THE SPIKE LIFE DIFFERENT?

This is the number one question. There are millions of diet plans out there. I know because it feels like I've tried them all, so what separates Spike Life from Diet A or Diet Z?

It's important that you know Spike Life was created by someone who has struggled with weight just like you. I lived through the pain and frustration of being overweight. *Spike Life* is written from the perspective of a man that went from morbidly obese to extremely fit. This is a book of sound scientific theory and real world results. *Spike Life* will show you the actual relationship of food, hormones, and metabolism, and how to swing the odds of success into your favor.

The truth is most diet and exercise plans negatively affect metabolism and hormones. This is one of the reasons why people who lose weight gain it back. Spike Life works in harmony with our hormones and body instead of against them. Another reason why the vast majority of dieters eventually regain the weight they lost is they are not in control and can't stick to their plans. Their diets are too restrictive or perhaps their exercise plan is too rigorous to maintain long term.

No one will ever claim Spike Life is too restrictive. This eating plan is effective without eliminating any food groups and without depriving you. The calorie goals for six days a week are sufficient and once a week you get a Spike Day where you will be able to indulge and enjoy all of the foods you love.

Exercise is important to our health and for a fit body. Unfortunately, exercise plans that exhaust you daily usually end when we can no longer keep pace. This is why the Spike Life plan only requires a minimum of one hour a week of actual exercise. However, I recommend increasing daily activity by walking and engaging in other types of recreation. Spikers are allowed to exercise more but by setting only a small weekly exercise goal, more people will be able to stick to it.

Spike Life is different!
- ▶ Enjoyable
- ▶ Maintainable
- ▶ Effective
- ▶ Puts you back in control

SPIKE LIFE PUTS YOU IN CONTROL

We are overweight for a reason. Most of us simply love to eat. Some people call this an excuse but it's the truth. When I would diet in the past I always felt like I had no control. Sure, I could choose what foods I put into my mouth, and I could choose to go to the gym. Yet I still had no control because despite my best efforts, it never netted me the long-term results I desired. Even when I was "perfect" and I felt like I did everything right, it still felt the scale had a mind of its own. I can't count the number of times I hit a weight-loss plateau in the past when I never changed a single factor. Frustration over the fact I couldn't control my weight led me to just want to give up. I didn't see the point of depriving myself and working my tail off in the gym if I wasn't improving.

Other times, I could only be "good" for so long—whether it was a feeling of impending doom, or the fact I could no longer keep my cravings at bay. I would lose control emotionally and eat the foods that I was trying so hard to give up. The guilt and remorse I'd feel afterward would only compound my emotional despair.

I wasn't in the driver's seat, food was controlling me!

This was my life before I started spiking. Spike Life put me in control over my cravings. By no longer depriving myself of the foods I craved and dictating when I was allowed to eat those foods, I seized back control over my life. The scale also responded and I lost over 100 lbs.

When we are not in control we are like a ticking time bomb, ready to go off at any moment. It's a stressful position to be in when we are afraid to leave our comfort zone. We may be presented with some food that's been on our minds for days. Even if we try to say "no," we may feel pressure from a friend, or that devil on your shoulder saying, "Come on, one bite won't hurt you." The truth is one bite of anything won't hurt your weight loss efforts, but it can affect you emotionally. When food is in control, we struggle with the guilt and remorse afterward and it leaves us feeling like a failure. Some of us punish ourselves by heading to the gym for an hour of cardio and drastically cutting calories. Some of us just give up, and give in. This emotional roller coaster does far more damage than the food could possibly have caused. Yet this is what happens when we are feeling deprived and not in control.

In living the Spike Life, you will chose when you "jump off the wagon" instead of suffering a fall or slip. You will control when you indulge and what you eat. Remorse will no longer be an issue because Spike Days are planned and effective. As an added bonus, you will find the foods you love will actually taste even better without guilt sprinkled on top. When you don't feel deprived and you know that within a few days you can eat anything you want, you will feel the power of control back in your life. You won't fear leaving your comfort zone because you can easily say "no thank you" to anything, and instead, plan and have it on your Spike Day.

Spike Life isn't just about Spike Day

Spike Life isn't just about Spike Day. To live the Spike Life to its full potential, you need to know how to make good food choices the other six days. This book is going to show you what kinds of foods are weight loss allies and which foods we should reserve for Spike Days. Our allies are foods that provide us with nutrition, boost metabolism, and make us feel fuller so we can be satisfied with fewer calories. I believe that the most important aspect of weight loss is "calories-in versus calories-out" and not the types of food that provide those calories. You could potentially "cheat" during the week and lose weight as long as you've stayed within your calorie range. The only problem is the foods we eat on Spike Day are often very calorie dense, and they don't provide us much relief from hunger or give our body the nutrition it needs. The easiest way to stay within your calorie range is to eat a balanced diet of healthy food. These types of foods are also often very nutritionally dense so that we are able to have stable energy and allow our body to recover from exercise. I prefer to save the calorie dense foods for my Spike Day when I'm able to eat them guilt free and my calorie goal is much higher than the other six days. I have a mental switch that is set to *healthy food* during the week, and on Spike Day, I flip the switch to *fun food*.

Spike Lifestyle Basics:
- ▶ Each day, stay within your calorie range to create a weekly caloric deficit
- ▶ Six days a week: the calorie range
- ▶ Spike Day once a week
- ▶ Use the Spike Life Food Pyramid for meal planning
- ▶ Eat foods high in protein and fiber at every meal
- ▶ Eat when you're hungry and not on an hourly schedule
- ▶ Prioritize resistance training for exercise
- ▶ Be more active daily, walk 10,000 steps daily
- ▶ Sleep 7-8 hours a night
- ▶ Refer to the section on *Troubleshooting Your Cravings* when you are struggling

CHAPTER 2

THE CURRENT STATE OF OBESITY

You don't have to read the statistics to know that obesity is perhaps the biggest health epidemic our generation and our children's generation will face. According to the World Health Organization (WHO), there are more than 1 billion overweight adults in the world and the number is quickly growing. While the statistics below are quite depressing, I want you to know that spiking can change everything. I want you to join me in the 5% of people who lose weight and keep it off forever!

Sad and scary statistics on obesity

- In the U.S. today, two out of every three adults are overweight
- The Centers for Disease Control and Prevention (CDC) predicts that by 2020, nearly 75% of all Americans will be overweight
- The percentage of obese adults has doubled in the past 30 years
- Less than one third of American adults are at a healthy weight
- More than 45-50 million Americans admit to dieting each year
- Americans spend $1-2 billion a year on weight loss products
- On average, obese people spend an extra $1,429 on healthcare costs
- The Centers for Disease Control and Prevention reports that more than 66% of Americans, two out of three people, is *actively* trying to either lose weight or maintain their current weight
- 95% of people who lose weight will gain it all back or more *(Colorado State University Extension food and nutrition)*
- Despite major efforts from consumers, governments, and thousands of diet programs and centers, obesity is still rising

Obesity isn't just an issue in America, it's a worldwide epidemic. Obesity rates are rising dramatically across the globe, and even though governments and consumers spend billions of dollars to remedy the situation, it continues to get worse.

The "Perfect Storm" for Obesity

We live in a time where food is abundant and we no longer need to be active to survive or work. Most of our jobs are sedentary yet very stressful.

These and many other factors are working against us

- We're stressed and busy

- ► We lead sedentary lifestyles
- ► There is cheap and convenient food on every corner
- ► We don't make or have no time to exercise
- ► Our body strikes back when we attempt to lose weight

Many people who are overweight are not lazy and they do care

I hate the common stereotypes that all overweight people are lazy and simply lack the willpower to say no. That stereotype is so far from the truth and so personal that few other statements cause me as much anger.

Well, I guess I do have to take some credit for my gluttony. I do love to eat food, especially the really calorie dense ones like ice cream and donuts, but I'm not lazy and I do care.

The reason I have a hard time saying no to "bad foods" is my brain is hardwired to crave them, so of course I love them. They taste amazing because my brain tells me they do. Calorie dense food means plenty of energy for my body without my metabolism having to expend lots of energy to process it. It's premium fuel and our brain is crazy for it! It's only natural that you and I crave those foods.

Remember, it's NOT your fault you are overweight, and there's no time for guilt while living the Spike Life. I know it's not your fault because it also wasn't mine. In the past I wasn't in control and I didn't know that my constant dieting was making my cravings worse.

We try to lose weight

We spend our hard-earned money trying to lose weight and live healthier lives but we are still overweight. The government spends money in the billions to fix the obesity epidemic and they have yet to find a true solution. Nothing proposed has ever improved the state of obesity. In fact, it's just getting worse.

What the experts don't understand is we are not statistics. Thin people don't have greater willpower than us. We are not all lazy. Being overweight does not make us less of a person than thin people, and actually, we are really more of a person. We are individual people with true emotional and physical connections to food. We love food just as much as we want to be thin. We are mentally hard-wired in a way that cannot be fixed by money or even desire. This is a place and time where all of the factors that cause obesity are at their peak, the perfect storm. The planets are all aligned and we are trapped by their gravitation pull. None of us wants to be overweight. We didn't choose these bodies or our genetics. We try to do what the experts tell us and it doesn't work. This is because those weight loss plans were not designed for you and me. We need to be allowed to live the way we are hard-wired or we will fail at losing weight long-term. Spike Life is for you and me. This is the way to improve your body on the outside while staying the person you are on the inside.

BODY MASS INDEX

BMI is used by doctors and researchers to determine if you are overweight or obese.

According to the CDC, obesity is a person with a BMI (Body Mass Index) of 30.0 or above.

Body Mass Index is determined by using a weight and height calculation. BMI is used because it's non-invasive, easy to track, and for many people, it correlates with their amount of body fat. It is very important to note that athletes and those with more muscular frames can be in the overweight/obese BMI range with a healthy amount of body fat.

BODY MASS INDEX (BMI) CHART												
WEIGHT	140	150	160	170	180	190	200	210	230	230	240	250
5'0"	27	29	31	33	35	37	39	41	43	45	47	49
5'3"	25	27	28	30	32	34	36	37	39	41	43	44
5'6"	23	24	26	28	29	31	32	34	36	37	39	40
5'9"	21	22	24	25	27	28	30	31	33	34	36	37
6'0"	19	20	22	23	25	26	27	29	30	31	33	34
6'3"	18	19	20	21	23	24	25	26	28	29	30	31

(HEIGHT is the vertical axis label for the rows.)

My opinion on BMI

I have called BMI "Bad Misleading Information" in the past, but I do believe BMI is a good general estimation of a person is overweight or obese. But it can also be extremely misleading for people who work out. At my heaviest recorded weight, I had a BMI of 42.4, which would put me in the "Extremely Obese" range. Today I'm a very healthy 215 lbs with only 9% body fat. My body fat percentage puts me in the very fit "athlete range," but at the same time my BMI is 27.6, which puts me in the "overweight" range for BMI.

This is where BMI is very misleading. Since BMI is simply a formula of one's height and weight, people with more lean body mass can be put in the "overweight" range while they are extremely healthy. Others may have extremely low lean body mass and be in the "normal" range for BMI, but have a high body fat percentage. BMI is the formula used for the research when we are told two out of three Americans are overweight. While a person with "muscle" listed as overweight is an error in these reports, I believe BMI is a useful tool for charting general population trends, but for Spike Life I would rather focus on body fat percentage and feeling amazing than to only care about weight on a scale and BMI.

Body fat percentage is more important than BMI

It's important to know your body fat percentage (bf%). I highly recommend you find your bf% when you start, and have it tested monthly. Body fat percentage is a much better gauge of progress then your weight on the scale. There may be weeks when you don't lose any weight on the scale, but at the same time, you burned away fat pounds. If you can accurately measure your body fat you, can separate your "good weight," lean body mass (LBM) and your "bad weight," fat pounds. Most of our pounds on the scale are lean body mass, and when we try to lose weight we don't want to lose any of it. You will learn later that lean body mass really drives our metabolism, and when we lose LBM our metabolism slows down. Many Spikers not only maintain their LBM while losing weight but they often increase it. So if you only look at the scale as a way of measuring progress, you may be disappointed at times when in reality, you should be celebrating.

BODY FAT PERCENTAGE CLASSIFICATIONS*		
CLASSIFICATION	**WOMEN (BF %)**	**MEN (BF %)**
ESSENTIAL FAT	10-12%	2-4%
ATHLETE	14-20%	6-13%
FIT	21-24%	14-17%
ACCEPTABLE	25-31%	18-25%
OBESE	32%+	25%+

American Council on Exercise

Ways to measure your body fat
- Skin fold calipers
- Bioelectrical impedance
- Hydrostatic (water displacement)
- Bod Pod
- Tape measure and weight formula

1. Skin Fold Calipers—Accuracy Score A-
Calipers are measuring tools available at most gyms and doctor's offices. Caliper body

fat testing measures skin folds on various body parts to calculate total body fat. It can be very accurate when measured by those with experience, but there is room for human error.

2. Bioelectrical Impedance—Accuracy Score B

This high-tech method is available at gyms, medical centers, and your bathroom. A small amount of harmless electrical current is delivered through the body to calculate total body water in lean tissue and muscle. Fat contains no water so body fat percentage is based on the difference between your body weight and lean tissue.

Results can be inaccurate if you are dehydrated or over-hydrated.

3. Underwater Body Fat Testing—Accuracy Score A+

This is a very accurate but expensive procedure. It is usually done at medical or university research facilities. The basic idea is that fat floats while bone and muscle sink. The person being measured is submerged into a water tank in a special chair with a weight belt attached to their waist. A technician repeats the procedure many times then calculates body density based on the difference between what your body weighs in air and water.

4. The Bod Pod—Accuracy Score A+

The Bod Pod is a cool egg-shaped chamber that is one of the most accurate ways to measure body fat. It is used by professional sports teams, hospitals, universities, and research centers. Tests can be expensive but they are also easier than underwater testing.

5. Tape Measure Formula—Accuracy Score B

This is the simplest way to accurately measure your body fat percentage. It can be done at home and all you need is a scale and a tape measure. It's not as accurate as other methods but it does give you a good estimate and a number to work with.

Try the tape measure formula at home

- ▶ Step 1—Weigh yourself first thing in the morning
- ▶ Step 2—Perform your circumference measurements with a tape measure that uses inches
  - ▶ Both men and women measure the circumference of their waist at the navel.
  - ▶ Women must also measure the circumference of their hips, forearm, and wrist. Measure your hips and forearm at their largest point. Take your wrist measurement at its thinnest point.
- ▶ Step 3—Calculate your lean body mass for both men and women

▶ Step 4—Convert your lean body mass to your body fat percentage

> LEAN BODY MASS FORMULA FOR MEN
> LBM = (weight x 1.082) - (waist circumference x 4.15) + 94.42

Example:

Luke weighs 215 lbs., and he has 34-inch waist. These measurements give Luke a lean body mass of:

(215 x 1.082) - (34 x 4.15) + 94.42 = 185.95 (LBM)

> LEAN BODY MASS FORMULA FOR WOMEN
> LBM = (weight x 0.732) - (waist circumference x 0.157)
> - (hip circumference x 0.249) + (forearm circumference x 0.434)
> + (wrist circumference / 3.14) + 8.987

Example:

Leia weighs 130 lbs, and she has a 30-inch waist, 36-inch hips, 8-inch forearm circumference, and a 6-inch wrist circumference. These measurements give Leia a lean body mass of:

(130 x 0.732) - (30 x 0.157) - (36 x 0.249) + (8 x 0.434) + (6 / 3.14) + 8.987 = 95.85 LBM

> CONVERT YOUR LEAN BODY MASS TO YOUR BODY FAT PERCENTAGE
> BF% = ((total weight - lean body mass) / total weight) x 100

Example:

Luke weighs 215 lbs and has 185.95 lbs of LBM which calculates to a BF% of:

((215 - 185.95) / 215) x 100 = 13.5% body fat

HOW OFTEN SHOULD I MEASURE MY BODY FAT PERCENTAGE?

I recommend measuring your BF% at least once a month; you could also do it weekly. Watching your BF% drop will provide you extra motivation on your journey. If you don't have access to these testing procedures, there is an easy-to-use body fat calculator at Spikelifebook.com

CHAPTER 3

WHY DIETING DOES NOT WORK

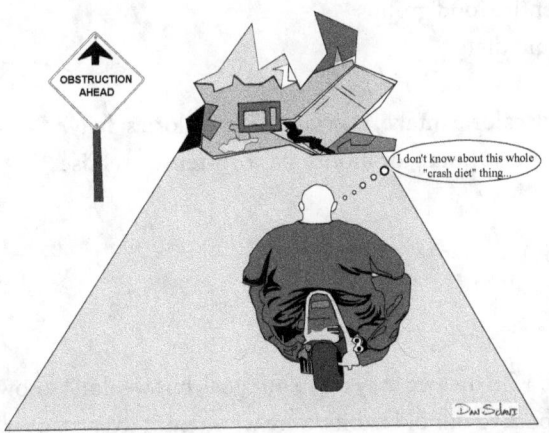

This chapter is about how many of us perceive dieting and exercise, and why most of us gain weight back after we lose it.

WE'RE INSANE—DIETS DON'T WORK!

I am not insane, but desperation to lose weight and be fit caused me to act like I was insane. Albert Einstein defined insanity as, "Doing the same thing, over and over again, and expecting different results." When I felt motivated I would exercise and diet to lose weight and within a few months I'd gain the weight back. I would then coast for a bit until I grew dissatified and motivated enought to start a new diet, then I would lose the weight again and eventually regain all I had lost. I did this over and over again, and for some reason each time I did this I expected that I would keep the weight off for good. I was, by his definition, acting insane.

I was the typical "yo-yo dieter." The problem wasn't that I didn't know how to lose weight. I just didn't know how to keep it off. Since you are reading this book, I'd expect that you too have acted "insane" just like I did in the past.

Fad Diets

The first mistake we commit when we decide to lose weight is choosing the plan. We look for the easiest way to lose as much weight as possible and in the shortest amount of time. It could be the latest low calorie fad diet that some big movie star or future queen just did to lose 20 lbs in a month, or an insane exercise routine that requires us to sweat for hours a day. Or it's a new miracle weight loss pill, patch, or powder we sprinkle on food. These fads do not work, and while we know better, we still fall for these schemes because our desperation to be thin makes us temporarily insane.

Common Dieting Fads
▶ Eliminate entire food groups
▶ Juice or liquid diets
▶ Fasting
▶ Severely low calorie intake, less than 1,200 calories daily
▶ Extreme exercise hours, or more a day of intense exercise
▶ Drugs
▶ Pills
▶ Patches
▶ Powders

When we choose a fad diet we may reach our goal, but we don't know what to do next. So we slowly go back to our old habits. Sure we attempt to carry over some of our new healthy choices, but most of us just can't stick to it. We have been food deprived and working hard for so long that we've just had enough. Not to mention that our motivation is no longer the same as it was early on when we were striving for our goal. Eventually it snowballs and we gain all the weight back. Then we become motivated once again and then we're on to the next big diet fad. This is the life of a constant dieter.

Although we celebrate success when we lose weight on a diet, true success happens when we are able to stick to our new lifestyle and keep the weight off for good. When we choose the fast and extreme path to weight loss, we set ourselves up for inevitable failure. Weight gain tends to happen when we believe that dieting is simply a quick fix for a lifelong weight control problem.

In search of the Magic Weight Loss Pill
The magic weight loss pill is like modern day snake oil that preys on our desperation. No one has ever wanted a magic weight loss pill more than me. It would be amazing if a single pill could make us thin, but I wouldn't hold my breath. There are diet pills available, but these diet pills will never on their own make you thin. The honest truth is there isn't a magic pill and there never will be. There is no magic in gaining weight either. Sometimes it may feel that way, because at times nothing seems to work as if there was some evil magic trapping us in our overweight bodies. Once you understand the science behind metabolism and how our body adapts to dieting, it will all make sense. Losing weight will no longer seem like a game of chance, hope, and despair. This knowledge is power, and with this knowledge you will finally have control over your life and your weight. There's no need for snake oil, just patience and faith.

Choosing the right weight loss plan

I tell people all the time that whether or not they choose my weight loss plan, they need to choose a plan that they could follow long term.

The plan you choose needs to become your new lifestyle. One reason why the majority of people who lose weight gain it back is because they didn't stick to their diet plan after they lost weight. Either they saw their diet as a quick fix or their diet was too restrictive to follow as a long-term lifestyle.

STOP THE INSANITY!

If we approach diets as a "quick fix" then that is exactly what they will be. You may lose weight, but you will almost surely gain it back like most people do. To become one of the few who have not gained the weight back you need to find a weight loss plan that you can follow long-term; a lifestyle, not a diet. This why diets that eliminate an entire food group, like "no-carb" diets, or worse, the extremely low calorie diets, also known as VLCD, that restrict our daily calories to 800 or even 500 calories, are doomed to fail us long-term.

The good news is you can lose weight without feeling deprived, and you can lose weight without having to exercise for hours a day. You can lose weight the spike way.

What does work:

- ▶ Motivation & Commitment
- ▶ Knowledge
- ▶ Commitment
- ▶ Control
- ▶ Patience
- ▶ Partner Up!
- ▶ Logging in a food journal
- ▶ Enjoying the Journey

You need to be motivated and committed

When I'm motivated I will make it happen, I'm committed. I bet you are the same way. Most of us are extremely motivated at the beginning of a weight loss plan. The problem is our motivation usually dies off as we go. It may be our plan loses its novelty or we become bored with it. Trust me, with my ADHD, I understand wanting to jump around and try the next great thing. The problem is this is the nasty cycle of yo-yo dieting. I think we do lose motivation and become bored when our results aren't what they used to be. We also may feel deprived from giving up our favorite foods. This is what happens when we try crash diets: those diets where we eliminate entire food groups and completely give up the foods we love. In the beginning, these diets may provide high amounts of weight loss from consuming extremely low amounts of calories. Eventually our brain catches on to our game and our metabolism slows down, making it harder to lose weight. At the same time cravings increase significantly and our motivation crashes along with the crash diet.

Spike Life will keep your motivation strong, because you can lose weight and never feel deprived. When you're motivated you're committed.

You need knowledge

You will learn most of the knowledge you need to manage a healthy weight in this book, but I don't want you to stop there. I encourage you to read other diet books, fitness blogs, message boards, and articles. You can learn something new each and every time. It might be a new workout, recipe, or tip that you can use. This is the most important knowledge you will ever learn since it can improve your life and maybe even save it. I want you to become passionate about your health, and once you do you will no doubt succeed. Make sure you keep in the mind the 10 Diet Myths so you can look past the bad information.

You need patience

We didn't gain weight in a day and we won't lose it in a day either. It is much better to lose one to three pounds a week than to crash-diet and attempt to lose more. Remember the Tortoise and the Hare! Losing weight at a slower but steady pace will greatly improve your odds of keeping the weight of forever and winning the race. You need to be patient and have faith in this plan, understand your calories in versus calories out numbers that you will learn later in this book. Then you know that even if the scale is having an "off" day, you were right where you needed to be. Water weight fluctuates often. One week the scale can show zero pounds lost and then the next week 4 lbs lost. When this happens, chances are you lost 2 lbs of fat both weeks, but the first week water weight hid the results on the scale.

Having a partner helps you succeed

Having a friend go on this journey with you increases your odds of success. Women who exercise with a partner lose an average of 10 lbs more than those that work out alone. Having someone hold you accountable will help you stay on track. With a partner you can motivate and support each other during more difficult times.

Avoid people who try to sabotage your goals. There is the theory that *misery loves company* and this can be very true while dieting. Some people are intimidated by your commitment, and instead of joining you they may try and bring you down to their level. You deserve positive reinforcement from your friends and family; confront them if they aren't providing you with that.

Keep a food journal

In a recent study by the Kaiser Permanente Center for Health Research, participants who kept food journals lost almost *double the weight* of those who did not log their calories.

Journaling your calories is extremely important to making and maintaining your progress. This is the *history and action plan of your diet*, and if there's a problem it will show in your logs. I've had many clients realize that they were eating too little or too much after they starting logging their meals. It also lets you know what you can have for dinner or a nighttime snack. I know it's tedious but this is too important to not take the time to do it. If you are computer savvy, there are many free online food journaling sites that make searching and logging meals extremely easy. Many of them also have smart phone apps so you can stay on track while away from home.

Enjoy the Journey!

Spike Life is the most enjoyable way to lose weight that you will ever find. Spikers love this program because they have control, they don't feel deprived, and they get results. You have the amazing opportunity to be *born again*, a fresh start, and redefine yourself as the person you want to be. This journey is full of self-discovery and when you reach your goal you will be filled with new confidence and the feeling that you can do anything. Trust me, you can do anything!

COMMON DIETING MYTHS

Common Dieting Myths

1. Eat six small meals a day to increase metabolism
2. Eat breakfast like a king, lunch like a prince, and dinner like a pauper
3. Don't eat before going to sleep
4. All extra calories are stored as fat
5. You can't go back to eating clean after a cheat day
6. High protein diets make you fat
7. Do aerobic exercise and not strength training to burn fat
8. Women who lift weights become "bulky" like men
9. We burn more body fat in the "Fat Burning Zone" for cardio
10. Cholesterol is bad for you

Diet Myth #1

EAT SIX SMALL MEALS A DAY TO INCREASE METABOLISM

This is one of the most common dieting myths, and one that I believed in for a long time. I lived by this rule only because it was hammered into my head for many years.

The truth is recent studies have proved that meal frequency has zero effect on metabolism. That's right, whether you eat six small meals, three larger meals, or one huge meal, if the calories are equal, then they all have the same metabolic effect. The reason why is our body has to metabolize every calorie we consume and it doesn't matter when we have them. For me, learning that six meals a day had no added benefits for metabolism was extremely liberating. I no longer felt the need to force myself to consume calories every two to three hours, and instead I could just eat when I feel hungry. There are times I push the hours between my meals out longer because I'm not hungry. If I'm hungry then I eat, if not then I wait until I am. This makes sticking to a daily calorie goal much easier. If I was eating a meal every few hours even when I wasn't hungry, I would often find myself hungry later but without any calories left in my goal for me to eat. For you this new rule gives you freedom to decide when you want to eat. You can still consume six small meals if you want, but you no longer have to.

New Diet Rule: Eat when you are hungry and stick to a calorie range

Diet Myth #2

BREAKFAST LIKE A KING, LUNCH LIKE A PRINCE, AND DINNER LIKE PAUPER

This old rule is linked to the meal frequency myth. What really matters is overall calories for the day. It only makes sense that you could spread those calories over the day any way you want. I know we are told that we should eat a large breakfast for energy, but if we are overweight we have plenty of energy stored on our body as calories in our fat cells. If we don't consume enough calories to fulfill our energy needs, our metabolism burns body fat to make up the difference. I actually live in direct contradiction of this myth. I prefer to have a high protein and lower calorie breakfast. Protein boosts my metabolism, and by not consuming a high carbohydrate breakfast, I lessen the impact on my blood sugar in the morning. It's called breakfast because we are literally *breaking our fast* from overnight, and carbohydrates have a larger effect on blood glucose levels and then insulin when we are in a fasted state. When we spike our blood glucose levels we are given a short term energy boost, but then it usually crashes soon after, causing us to be hungry yet again. High calorie breakfast cereals are one of the worst choices first thing in the morning, while bacon and eggs are a great choice because they keep blood glucose stable and keep us feeling full and satisfied for hours. My largest meal every day is dinner. That's when I'm the hungriest and I have the most time to prepare a healthy meal. I've adjusted my daily meal plan to allow for extra calories at night. With Spike Life we are given a daily calorie goal and you are able to adjust the daily meal plan to fit the way you want to eat.

New Diet Rule: Your largest meal can be at any time of the day.

Diet Myth #3

DON'T EAT BEFORE GOING TO SLEEP

Let me clear the air and assure you that you are not a Gremlin; if you eat before bed or even after midnight you will not turn into a fat-storing monster. Our body doesn't magically store body fat after a certain hour. We burn calories through metabolism 24 hours a day, and even though our metabolism dips a bit while we sleep, the difference is minimal. I think going to bed hungry is the one of the worst choices we can make. While our body rests, our brain is extremely active while we sleep. Our brain feeds mainly off of glucose and it needs many of those calories at night. Since we are technically fasting for several hours our brain can become stressed with the lack of available energy and begin converting muscle to glucose to provide the needed fuel. This issue is compounded when we stop eating hours before we go to sleep. I know of many people who were told to not eat after 7pm, and that just adds several more hours to their nighttime fast. I personally eat a healthy snack right before I go to bed, even it that is after midnight, and I have yet to turn into a Gremlin.

⚠ New Diet Rule: Never go to bed hungry

Diet Myth #4

ALL EXCESS CALORIES ARE STORED AS FAT

Many of us are afraid that if we ever overeat, all of the excess calories will just make us fatter. This is false. Our body stores excess calories in our muscle and liver glycogen first, and when those stores are full, the remaining calories are converted and stored as fat. You will learn more about energy or calorie storage later in this book. It is nice to know that we have a buffer between excess calories and fat storage.

⚠ New Diet Rule: Overeating once in a while doesn't make you fat

Diet Myth #5

YOU CAN'T GO BACK TO EATING HEALTHY AFTER A CHEAT DAY

I was always afraid to have a cheat day when I was trying to lose weight, because I thought if I "gave in" I wouldn't be able to stop. This is a huge topic in this book and you will learn that cravings have less to do with willpower and more to do with our brain and hormones. Physical cravings are not something we can consciously control, and as far as this myth is concerned, the opposite is true. When we deprive ourselves of the foods we love and restrict calories, our cravings increase significantly. When we cheat once in a while, our physical cravings actually decrease and we are able to make better food choices.

⚠ New Diet Rule: Occasionally enjoying your favorite foods on a diet

helps eliminate both mental and physical cravings.

Diet Myth #6

HIGH PROTEIN DIETS MAKE YOU FAT

This couldn't be further from the truth. Protein actually helps us lose more weight because it has high-level satiety, boosts metabolism, and helps to build lean muscle mass. According to studies in the *American Journal of Clinical Nutrition,* when protein is increased, dieters reported greater satisfaction, less hunger, and greater weight loss. I believe this myth started because high protein diets are wrongly associated with high fat diets, but you can have high protein without being high in dietary fat. Spike Life is a high protein diet when compared to the average American diet, but in reality, it's a very balanced diet of proteins, carbohydrates, and fats.

New Diet Rule: High protein diets help you lose weight

Diet Myth #7

DO AEROBIC EXERCISE AND SKIP STRENGTH TRAINING TO BURN FAT

When we decide to lose weight we picture hours a day of sweating on a cardio machine or joining an aerobics class to burn body fat. Some people are actually afraid to strength train because they think this will lead to gaining weight and not the ultimate goal of weight loss. The truth is aerobics do not burn more body fat than weight lifting. Both types of exercise burn extra calories while we are exercising, but the difference is what happens post-exercise. When we finish our cardio our metabolism will eventually come back down to normal and our reward was simply burning X amount of calories. When we strength train we tear muscle fibers that our body has to repair while we rest and recover. This is an extra job for our metabolism, and the process of rebuilding muscle tissue increases our metabolism while it's in the recovery process. Another bonus is added muscle has a direct effect on our resting metabolism. The more muscle we have, the higher our metabolism. In conclusion: aerobics burn calories only while we exercise, while strength training burns calories while we exercise and while we recover, and increases our resting metabolism when we become stronger. Strength training has a 3-1 advantage over aerobics for fat-burning. As far as gaining weight, the process of bulking up requires excess calories. You will not gain weight while you are in a caloric deficit. So there should be no fear of weight gain while we strength train and restrict calories.

New Diet Rule: Lifting weights is a great way to burn body fat

Diet Myth #8

WOMEN WHO LIFT WEIGHTS BECOME "BULKY" LIKE MEN

This is one of the worst myths out there since it stops some women from doing one of the best fat-burning exercises available: strength training. Women are not hormonally designed to build muscle like men, it's just not possible. Muscle on women makes them look leaner and also boosts their metabolism. Strength training should be a priority for women who want to lose weight and not avoided.

New Diet Rule: Women who lift weights are lean and tone

Diet Myth #9
WE BURN MORE BODY FAT IN THE "FAT-BURNING ZONE" FOR CARDIO
It is true that we burn a higher percentage of body fat in the "fat-burning zone," but we burn more overall calories per minute in higher intensity zones. You should be able to burn more actual body fat calories at a high intensity for 30 minutes than a low intensity. Expending more calories also leads to increased fat burning by creating a larger daily caloric deficit.

New Diet Rule: You burn more fat calories with intense exercise than in the "Fat-Burning Zone"

Diet Myth #10
CHOLESTEROL IS BAD FOR YOU
Cholesterol is a vital part of each one of our cells in our bodies. We need cholesterol, it's essential to our health. It can help us lose weight because it's precursor to the anabolic hormones that help us build muscle. Testosterone in males drops when cholesterol is too low. LDL and HDL are lipoproteins; they are fats combined with proteins. Some LDL or low density lipoproteins can squeeze through artery linings and become rancid, causing inflammation, but then HDL or high density lipoproteins sweep in and carry them away. HDL is extremely important for our health as it cleans our arteries of stagnate cholesterol and triglycerides. Our ratio of HDL to LDL is far more important than a cholesterol number. Most natural fats increase our HDL numbers while hydrogenated fats and carbohydrates raise triglycerides and LDL numbers.

New Diet Rule: Natural fats and cholesterol increase healthy HDL cholesterol

SPIKE LIFE RULES OF WEIGHT LOSS
Knowing the truth allows us to create a plan

▶ Be in control of your food and life

- ▸ Stick to a daily calorie range
- ▸ Eat when you are hungry
- ▸ Have protein and fiber with every meal
- ▸ Keep your blood sugar stable
- ▸ Never go to bed hungry
- ▸ Have a Spike Day once a week after days of calorie restriction
- ▸ Men and women should incorporate strength training to burn more body fat
- ▸ Be active and walk daily
- ▸ Never feel guilty and strive to be optimistic
- ▸ Find a partner to support your weight loss journey
- ▸ Don't be afraid of natural fats and cholesterol

PART II

CALORIES IN VERSUS CALORIES OUT

Key Terms:

Energy—In relation to weight loss, energy is calories. We use a *calorie* to measure the energy in food and the energy we expend. Energy Balance and Calorie Balance is the same thing.

Law of Thermodynamics—The unbreakable rule of calories in versus calories out equals energy burned or stored, or fat loss versus fat gain.

Glycogen—A stored form of glucose in our liver and our muscles used to stabilize blood sugar levels and provide energy to our muscles.

Thermic Effect of Food—The metabolic boost from calories we consume.

CHAPTER 4

THE LAW OF THERMODYNAMICS

The Law of Thermodynamics is the rule of *calories in versus calories out* is equal to *weight loss or weight gain*. It's a law we can't break, but when we diet our body finds ways to bend the law to keep us overweight. Spike Life takes this challenge head on, and bends the law back in our favor.

THE LAW OF THERMODYNAMICS

As it pertains to diets, The Law of Thermodynamics is the law of *calories in versus calories out*, and like any of our natural laws, it can't be broken. This is the reason why we lose weight on all types of diets or we gain weight when we quit going to the gym.

One side of the scale is the energy (calories) we bring in to our body and the other side is the energy (calories) we expend. It's very similar to a car; we put energy, gasoline, into a car and the car then burns that energy to get from one place to the next. If the gasoline isn't totally used up then it's stored in the tank until the next time we drive.

Once we disrupt the balance of either side of the thermodynamic scale by either eating too many calories, or too few, we create an energy imbalance. We then store excess energy and gain weight, or we burn stored energy and lose weight. This may be elementary to you, but it is very important that this law is fully understood and respected. Spike Life works within this law and any program that tells you that you can lose weight despite your caloric balance is not being honest with you.

Obey the Law

Now you may be confused because you thought that this was the book that said you can eat the foods you love and lose weight. Spike Life is about living the spike lifestyle, and Spikers should indulge one day every week on Spike Day. In fact, the goal of Spike Day is actually to consume a surplus of calories for one day. I know I said that the Law of Thermodynamics tells us that excess calories are stored in our body. I am not contradicting myself. It is beneficial to long term results to break the constant use of stored energy and actually store some energy. This should be done once every week. This is where the "magic" of spiking happens and why this program is extremely successful for long term results.

Spike Life focuses on the big picture of health and fitness; this isn't a program designed to help you lose 20 lbs in two weeks. If that is your goal then you have the wrong book. This lifestyle is about living a full and amazing life by losing weight without feeling deprived. This includes having the best of both worlds; the body you want and enjoying the foods you love. You no longer have to choose one or the other. While Spike Day is a tremendous mental break, the purpose of having one is actually to help you lose weight.

One day of overeating (Spike Day) when it follows six days of calorie restriction, will not make you fat. Do you think one day of eating perfect compensates for six days of eating bad? Of course not!

Spike Life bends the Law of Thermodynamics by not allowing our body to become accustomed to a lower calorie amount. This trick maximizes our body's potential to burn more fat for energy. As an additional bonus, most of the excess calories you consume on Spike Day will not be stored as fat but as glycogen. You will learn about the importance of glycogen and how it actually helps us get leaner later.

CHAPTER 5

ENERGY BALANCE

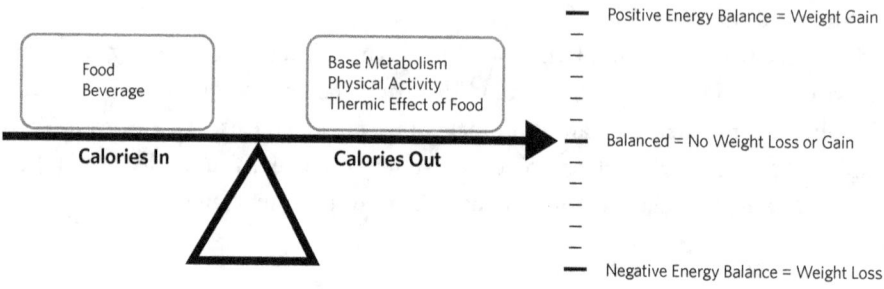

In this chapter I will teach about energy balance as it pertains to weight loss and weight gain. When I talk about energy, I'm referring to calories. Calories are the way we measure energy in our food and the fuel we use to make us move and function.

The Hormonal Weight Loss Battle

Insulin the "Fat-Storing Hormone" Vs. Glucagon the "Fat-Burning Hormone"

Insulin and glucagon are the hormones in our body responsible for storing energy and burning stored energy. These two hormones are like night and day. They are both produced in our pancreas but they cannot coexist at the same time. Glucagon is the fat-burning hormone, when there isn't enough available energy from our diet. Glucagon creates the energy we need by converting our fat and glycogen stores into energy. Insulin is the exact opposite. Insulin is the hormone that is released when we consume calories and is responsible for storing excess calories into our glycogen stores and fat cells. Insulin is highly sensitive to blood sugar levels. One of the ways to negate the negative attributes of insulin is by keeping our blood sugar stable by eating less refined carbohydrates and choosing foods that have a low Glycemic Load (GL).

It's important to note that insulin isn't all bad and glucagon isn't all good. Insulin is extremely important to building muscle, and at times, glucagon can burn our muscle tissue for energy. Building lean muscle is very important to long term success because of the effect it has on resting metabolism.

In living the Spike Life we want to maximize the positives and minimize the negatives effects of insulin and glucagon.

To get the maximum effect from Insulin:
▶ Keep our blood sugar stable
▶ To keep our blood sugar stable, we have fiber and protein with every meal

to slow the digestion of food
- ▶ Never have a high sugar or starch food on an empty stomach
- ▶ Immediately after a workout have a whey protein shake
- ▶ Eat a balanced meal within an hour after working out

To get the maximum effect from Glucagon:
- ▶ Keep our blood sugar stable to maintain low insulin levels
- ▶ Don't force meals every 2-3 hours when we are not hungry
- ▶ Never go to bed hungry
- ▶ Eat a high protein and fiber diet

POSITIVE ENERGY BALANCE
Surplus of calories leads to energy storage

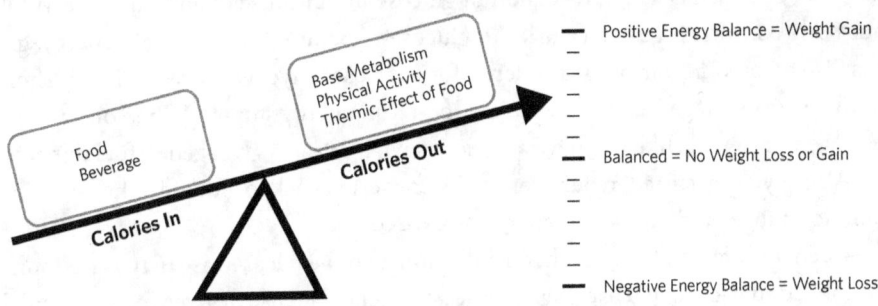

When we consume a surplus of calories we will store energy. There is no healthy way around this fact. It's really not anything to worry about if you have a day of overeating or even a larger meal. I look at the big picture to energy balance. I care about the long-term, not the short-term. We often store energy and burn stored energy all on the same day, so what really matters for true weight gain or weight loss is how we balance our calories over multiple days. Spike Life focuses on the "net deficit" of calories over a week.

Most of us are overweight because we eat too much on a regular basis. It's not because we eat great and then slip up for one day. It's nearly *impossible* for us to get fat with one bad day if we are eating at a caloric deficit the other days.

By following the Spike Life plan and being in a negative energy balance for six days, we would have to consume around 10,000 calories on Spike Day to gain even a pound of fat.

The truth is we only *get fat* when we overeat on a consistent basis.

Our body has two ways of storing excess energy

- ▶ Glycogen—Short-Term Energy Storage
- ▶ Body Fat—Long-Term Energy Storage

MUSCLE & LIVER GLYCOGEN

Some people simply assume that excess calories are stored as fat, and it's not totally true. I used to think that whenever I would overeat that it would just make me fatter. I also hear similar statements from health professionals and personal trainers, and it just isn't the entire truth. Excess calories are stored in our body, but what most people don't realize is that surplus energy is stored first in our liver and our muscles as glycogen. When our glycogen stores are at capacity, the calories left over are then converted to triglycerides and stored in our fat cells. In a sense, glycogen acts as a buffer between extra calories and stored body fat.

So what is glycogen?

Basically glycogen is a stored version of glucose in our muscles and our liver. While our body converts ingested calories to glucose to be used as immediate energy, glucose isn't stored in our body as energy for later use. Glycogen is what I call "short-term" energy storage while body fat is "long-term" energy storage. When our muscles needs energy quick, like when we are exercising, it releases glycogen to fuel our activity. Also, glycogen stored in our liver can be converted back to glucose to help stabilize our blood sugar and provide us energy as needed.

Stored body fat, on the other hand, takes longer to be released as energy and cannot be converted back to glucose. Making the availability and use of glycogen is extremely important to our body, and also one of the reasons why glycogen storage is higher priority to our body than storing body fat.

Glycogen is a hero to those who want to be fit. Besides blocking us from storing fat, it is also the best form of energy for exercise. We often feel lethargic and weak when we exercise with depleted glycogen, and full of energy and strong when glycogen is full. When we are able to exercise more efficiently, we also have better results. Also, liver glycogen helps us avoid the midday energy crash by helping to regulate our blood sugar levels. When we have more energy throughout the day, we are more effective at everything do. The problem with many people who are dieting is they have constantly low levels of stored glycogen. So they are always in a state of energy ups and downs, because they have to rely heavily on the calories they consume for daily energy to fuel their workouts.

One of the goals of living the Spike Life is to change our body from prioritizing the foods we eat for energy, and instead burn our stored energy. This is how we become a fat-burning machine. To do this we want to maximize our body's ability to store and use glycogen. When this is mastered, the process of losing weight and staying fit becomes much easier.

Spike Days are similar to "carbohydrate-loading"

This concept was easy for me to understand. Being an athlete, I remembered we would always do what the coach called "carb-loading" with a spaghetti dinner the night before our football games. Also, I have many friends who run marathons and glycogen is extremely important to runners. They would also do the same and eat a high amount of carbs and calories the day before their run. So you're probably thinking, "Hey, I'm not an athlete, and I'm definitely not running a marathon." Actually, you are an athlete, you're a *Spike Athlete*. Workouts are your sporting events and exercise will be your sport. By maximizing our ability to work out we will inevitably get in better and better shape. The mindset for exercise should not be "how many calories can I burn"; this just doesn't work. It has been well documented that simply burning calories through exercise doesn't work to make us thin. The mindset is instead on progression and improvement. If one week you can lift a weight for 9 reps, then the next week you want to do 10 reps. If you run for 10 minutes one week, then the next week it's 11 minutes. The calorie goals alone set in this book will initiate weight loss, and the exercise that I want to do will improve your strength and your muscle tone. In the long-term, your added muscle and strength will dramatically help you keep the weight off, and make exercise more fun. It's your event and not something you feel like you have to do. I hope you will begin to look forward to your workout instead of dreading it.

Glycogen improves exercise

I have learned through my experience that it is extremely difficult to exercise efficiently when our glycogen stores are depleted, but when glycogen has been maximized, my workouts went through the roof. When I first began "spiking" I began to see a pattern in my workouts. The day after my Spike Days, not only did I have more endurance, but my strength was also greatly enhanced. Living the Spike Life is a type of carbohydrate-loading program. For six days when I was in calorie restriction I was depleting my glycogen storage, and then on my Spike Day, which was a very high carbohydrate day, I was reloading my glycogen. So naturally, I made the day after my Spike Day my biggest workout; I began calling it my "After-Spike" workout. My after-spike workouts have allowed me to build muscle and become stronger while I was losing weight. This is an amazing benefit of spiking.

How many calories can we store as glycogen?

The amount of calories we store as glycogen varies from person to person. It depends on how many carbohydrates we consume, weight, and muscle mass of each person. Most untrained individuals can store between 100 grams to 150 grams of glycogen in their liver, and an additional 300 grams to 500 grams in their muscles. For many of us that is about 1,600 to 2,600 calories of stored energy as glycogen. Conditioned athletes are able to store a higher amount mainly in their muscles. The process of glycogen depletion and reloading is one of the ways that trains our body to increase glycogen storage. Glycogen is being used and stored every day, but when we are in calorie restriction, there are not many extra calories available to be stored. Because of this, athletic performance and exercise suffers.

After a Spike Day when we consciously consume a surplus of calories, our body is then able to restore glycogen and our workouts improve dramatically.

Have you ever felt dizzy or light-headed while you were working out?

This is exercise-induced hypoglycemia and it happens to all of us. Hypoglycemia is when your blood sugar has dropped because you didn't have enough calories. Your liver glycogen would have been able to pick up the slack and save you from feeling sick, but it was already depleted. I'm hoping you can see the importance of carbohydrates and glycogen to fitness. Carbohydrates get a bad rap when it comes to obesity, but they are not 100% bad. In fact, they play an important role in living the Spike Life.

Water Weight and Glycogen

With all of the good that comes with glycogen there is a little of the bad. If there is one negative to glycogen it is that when we store glycogen, we also store water. Typically our body stores three grams of water for every gram of glycogen. Since I'm a math guy I like to do the numbers; if you can store 400 to 650 grams of glycogen, you will also hold onto 1,200 to 1,950 grams of water or about 2.5 to 4 pounds.

Storing glycogen will increase our weight on the scale. For some people this is very hard to see—I know I am one of those people. When I've worked really hard and ate what I was supposed to, I expect to be rewarded by watching my weight decline on the scale. This is one of the reasons why the scale can be meaningless and why I warn people to not weight themselves after a Spike Day. True water weight can fluctuate daily, but our weight is definitely higher after we enjoy a Spike Day. Don't worry, though—we still burn body fat even when the scale may be up due to water weight gain. After spiking, water weight will be lost as we burn through glycogen during the upcoming week. Typically the water weight gain is gone 24-48 hours after spiking.

We focus on burning fat and not losing water weight

Glycogen and water weight is the big reason many people lose more weight the first week of a diet, specifically "low-carb" diets. We are able to lose four pounds of water weight much easier than burn four pounds of fat. So when someone loses six pounds in a week, we know that a big percentage of that weight loss was water, and as soon as they eat more carbohydrates, they will regain that water weight.

Water weight is insignificant, and it should not detract you from sticking to a plan that will get you to the ultimate goal. Look at it this way: water weight is lean body mass and lean body mass is what we want. The ultimate goal is to burn fat. The scale should never be the definitive judge because it's inconsistent. What truly matters is how you feel.

Spike Days increase our glycogen

If we are consuming a caloric deficit 6 days a week while increasing our activity level, our body is burning through our glycogen stores quickly. As glycogen depletes, our workouts become less effective. This is one reason why spiking is important. Spike Day is the ultimate "carb-loading" day; by restoring glycogen your workouts will improve dramatically. One day of spiking provides the fuel that you need to have intense workouts in the coming week. The day after my Spike Day I have the best workouts of the week. I call them my "After-Spike" or "Spiked" workouts. My endurance and strength are maxed out to their full potential and I quickly burn up my excess calories from the day before with a fun and intense workout.

> **!** SPIKE LIFE TIP
>
> To maximize the glycogen loading effect of spiking: Reduce your carbohydrate intake three days prior to your Spike Day, and then when you spike, eat 60% of your Spike Day calories from carbohydrates. This isn't a necessity for weight loss, but it further enhances the exercise benefits of spiking.

Glycogen Summary:

- Glycogen is a stored form of glucose
- Glycogen is stored in our muscles and liver
- Muscle glycogen fuels our muscles during activities
- Liver glycogen can help stabilize blood sugar
- We can increase our ability to store glycogen and maximize its effectiveness by depleting and reloading glycogen every week
- Carbohydrates and glycogen can improve athletic performance
- Your workout is your "athletic event"
- Excess calories are first stored as glycogen
- We store three grams of water for every gram of glycogen
- Water weight can be unpredictable and the scale is inconsistent

WHEN DO WE STORE BODY FAT?

Body fat is different than glycogen; while they are both ways our body is able to store energy, they serve different purposes. We are limited in the amount of glycogen we are able to store, but our bodies can store extreme amounts of calories in our fat cells. While storing energy in our fat cells has caused its own serious epidemic, we store body fat to help us survive when food is scarce. Body fat is really just a survival tool that our current lifestyles have turned into a monster. If we didn't have a way to store energy then we would die as soon as we didn't have enough food to eat. True, this isn't an issue for most of us living in the world today. Our body's ability to store fat has allowed the human race to survive through dire times of extreme famine. It may not be needed for you and me, but we are still hardwired the same way our ancestors were thousands of years ago.

Energy Storage by the Numbers

It is very important to understand the relationship between the calories we eat, expend, and store.

A pound of stored body fat is equal to 3,500 calories, but eating an excess 3,500 calories does mean we gained a pound of fat. Remember that excess calories are first stored as glycogen; the leftover calories, if there are any, will be stored as fat.

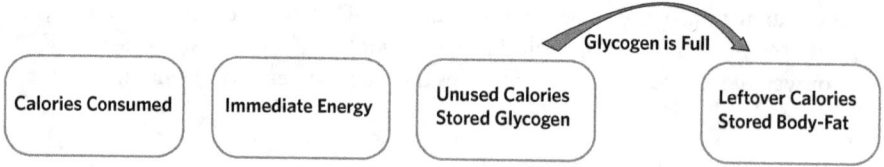

Gaining a pound on the scale doesn't necessarily mean we stored a pound of fat.

Water weight and glycogen are the X factors. Water weight can cause havoc on our bathroom scale, up two pounds one day and down two pounds the next. It's enough to drive anyone crazy, but you will know that as long as you are within your calorie range set in this book and staying active, then the scale becomes unimportant. You will know that in the long run your weight will go down and you can ignore the typical day to day scale fluctuations that inevitably happen.

STARVATION MODE

Chapter 6 is all about one of the most misunderstood and debated topics concerning weight loss: starvation mode. There's never been a doubt in my mind that it's real. I've personally experienced starvation mode in the past and I know how devastating it can be to one's weight loss goals. Science is now proving the existence of starvation mode and piecing together the details of how and why it happens.

WHAT IS STARVATION MODE?

Starvation mode is a hardwired survival adaptation in which our body undergoes several metabolic and mental changes to survive when we are not providing our body the calories it requires for daily functions. This begins when we are consistently in caloric restriction for several days or more and our brain is alerted to the imbalance. It sounds the panic alarm. Our cravings immediately increase to give us the drive to go and search out food. Then our metabolism is deregulated and slows down so we won't burn through our backup energy storage, body fat, as quickly as we would at normal speed.

The common response by those who doubt starvation mode's existence is: "We are not in a famine, and I'm obese with plenty of body fat to lose before I ever starve to death." Well true, most of us are not living in a time of famine; in fact, it's the exact opposite. But tell me, how does your brain know that? While the human brain is incredible, you really can't rationalize with its survival functions. The brain works on signals, responding to the environment our bodies are in. The most important function of our brain is our survival. So it is able to adapt in miraculous ways to keep us alive.

The truth is restricting calories to lose weight is like a self-induced famine. Our brain gets alerted that lots of stored energy is going out and we aren't replacing it. This is what triggers the alarm that we are on the path of starvation. Even if you are obese, this still can happen to you. It happened to me multiple times when I was over 300 lbs. It is perhaps the most frustrating side effect of dieting.

Don't worry about genetics

Losing weight is: 80% Diet -10% Exercise -10% Genetics

Some people believe that we all have a certain body fat "set point" and once we drop below that body fat percentage, starvation mode kicks in and we are stuck. I don't believe that at all. I was in starvation mode while dieting several times when I was over 300 lbs. Once I started spiking, starvation mode stopped. Since then I've been down to 200 lbs with single-digit body fat without ever being stuck at a plateau again. What the heck happened to my "set point"?

There is no genetic set point; you can be as ripped as you want. Truthfully, you can! Do you think I ever thought when I had a 46-inch waist that one day I'd have abs? No, if someone had told me that one day I'd have a six-pack, I would have actually laughed my weight off. Anything is possible when you have knowledge and faith.

I hate the talk of genetic set points. When you tell someone that they're stuck because they hit their genetic limit, why would they even try anymore? If that was true, I'd just give up, because what's the point of trying if I'm destined to be overweight? It's true that genetics do play a role, and some people do have it easier when it comes to being fit, but it's actually a small role. Our genetics are not a valid excuse for being overweight. If I can overcome my genetic trap, anybody can.

We don't have weight limits

Our brain doesn't take inventory of our fat storage; if it did then us humans should have a weight limit, but yet someone is always topping 1,000 pounds and breaking the world weight record. As far as starvation mode is concerned, it doesn't realize we have plenty of stored body fat. All it knows is that we are on a relentless trend of calorie restriction day after day. Our body, which strives for homeostasis, then adapts to put an end to our self-induced famine.

Caloric restriction is the cause of starvation mode

What causes starvation mode is simply calorie restriction for days, weeks, and months. As our metabolisms slows, it progressively gets more and more difficult to burn fat, until one day we hit the diet plateau. Then we either need to eat less and workout more, or risk gaining weight back. It's the *Nightmare on Diet Street* and starvation mode is more fiendish than Freddy Krueger.

Sure, none of us are literally starving, but how would our brain know the difference between major calorie restriction from a diet plan, and major calorie restriction from a real famine? Calorie restriction signals the survival alarm that a threat is near.

Starvation mode is the *metabolic response* to caloric restriction

Starvation mode is the misleading name for people like you and I, who are not literally starving, but we restrict calories to lose weight. It's more of a "metabolic response" to caloric restriction. When we say "starvation" we think of not eating or total food deprivation. While not eating will surely bring on this adaptation, so can dieting to a lesser extent. Starvation mode is triggered by several consecutive days of any amount of calorie restriction or caloric deficit. When we are consistently dipping into our energy reserves and not putting anything back, that is starvation as far as our bodies are concerned. Our body is literally eating itself for energy daily and that's a no-no for survival. This is why one of the first metabolic adoptions is increased hunger and cravings. Our brain is giving us a warning and trying to get us to eat more. If we ignore this warning more extreme changes are sure to come.

The idea of starvation mode has struck fear into many dieters. Sometimes they are coerced into eating more daily to keep starvation mode away even if they are not hungry. Starvation mode doesn't work that way. The truth is you could eat 1,000 or 1,500 calories every day for a month, but if you were burning 2,000 calories daily, both of those calorie goals could initiate starvation mode. I do believe the larger deficit will bring on faster and more extreme changes, but both could cause some metabolic adoptions because they both put you in caloric restriction.

STARVATION MODE MYTHS

Myth #1
MISSING A MEAL CAN CAUSE STARVATION MODE.
Wrong. It's about overall caloric balance and takes a sustained deficit of calories.

Myth #2
STARVATION MODE HAPPENS WHEN CALORIES ARE LOW FOR ONE DAY.
It gradually begins after several days of caloric restriction.

Myth #3
STARVATION MODE KICKS IN WHEN WE EAT FEWER THAN 1,200 CALORIES.
There is no "magic calorie" number for starvation mode; it's several consecutive days of any type of caloric restriction.

Myth #4
METABOLISM SLOWDOWN FROM STARVATION MODE CAN STOP YOU FROM LOSING WEIGHT COMPLETELY.
Often dieting plateaus are blamed solely on starvation mode. While a slower metabolism can contribute to it, usually water weight is the main culprit for day to day anomalies on the scale.

Starvation mode is real but there are many irrational fears about it. While the metabolism slowdown could not stop you from losing weight completely, I feel like any type of drop is unacceptable as it will make it more difficult to keep the weight off.

Signs you may be in Starvation Mode
- Increased food cravings
- Food obsession
- Fatigue

▶ Depression
▶ Anxiety
▶ Poor workout energy
▶ Decreased morning body temperature
▶ You're not losing as much weight as you should be, based on your calories consumed versus your total daily energy expenditure

My experience with starvation mode

The last time I was in starvation mode, my weight loss stalled, my workouts were losing intensity, and worst of all, I was having extreme food cravings. Not a simple, "I'd like to have a donut," but the kind of cravings that can drive a person crazy. I was more like "Give me a donut now or else!" It wasn't something my willpower could overcome. I was at a point of mental survival. I couldn't focus on many things other than eating and I knew I would eventually just give in to these temptations, like I had in the past. Knowing that it was inevitable, I took the bull by the horns and decided to plan my day of splurging. I wanted to maintain the control instead of food controlling me. This ended up as one of the greatest decisions of my entire life. It was the catalyst I needed to lose weight once and for all. At the time, I had no idea of the benefits that would come after. I just wanted to clear my head so I could function again.

After my success I researched what was happening and I learned that it wasn't a magical phenomenon. It was hormones that caused starvation mode and my Spike Day was rebalancing those hormones, specifically leptin.

LEPTIN: THE "ANTI-STARVATION" HORMONE

Leptin is a relatively new factor in the battle against obesity. It wasn't discovered until the 1990s. What researchers found was that leptin plays an integral role in monitoring our metabolism and our hunger. Leptin is found inside our fat cells. Its job is to tell our brain that we are full and satisfied when we eat. It functions in lean healthy adults without any issues. However, for those who are overweight and trying to lose weight, it plays mean and nasty tricks. When leptin is high, we are supposed to be satisfied and not feel the need to eat. However, when leptin is low it sends a warning signal to the brain that our body fat, which is our long-term energy supply, is quickly being used up. When this happens our hunger cravings greatly increase in an attempt to get us to search out food. Also, metabolism is slowed down so we will burn less body fat, thus prolonging the availability of our stored energy. Since our brain perceives this as a time of famine, we will survive longer on fewer calories, buying us more time until we feast.

It's amazing, really; our brain's number one job is survival. Our brain and body adapt in extraordinary ways to keep us alive in extreme situations.

In fact, people like you and me are more highly evolved. If there was ever to be a true time of famine, all of the perpetual thin people would be the first to go, leaving you and me to rule the world.

While it's a wonderful survival mechanism, it's extremely frustrating that our body fights back in such a way when we are just trying to improve our health. It does make complete sense when you think about it and when you've experienced it. Restricting calories is almost like a self-induced famine. How would our brain know the difference? It just senses the constant use of stored energy as a sign that there isn't enough to eat.

Research on Leptin

► Studies have shown that leptin levels can drop up to 50% in just seven days of calorie restriction.
► The researchers also found that the desire to eat doubled in response to calorie restriction. The participants reporting the greatest *increase in hunger* were those with the largest *decline in leptin*.

This is extraordinary news, because now we can have an action plan to deal with one of the biggest obstacles obstructing those trying to lose weight.

Some experts don't think it's possible, because they believe leptin declines when we are losing weight and we cross a personal "body fat threshold." *I don't think this is the whole story.*

Let's look at the numbers. The study showed in seven days of calorie restriction leptin can drop up to 50%. Well, on a good week some people lose only around one to three pounds of body fat, and that's on the high end.

Attributing the decline in leptin as simply a result of losing body fat, to me doesn't appear logical. I will use myself as an example; if leptin decline happens solely because we are burning up fat storage, how in the world could I have lost over 130 lbs of pure body fat? I should have no leptin left! I should be eating everything in sight and my metabolism should be so low that I wouldn't be able to get out bed.

Leptin decline does not simply happen because we cross a personal body fat threshold. Is it logical to think that the people in the study who had a 50% decline in leptin crossed their body fat threshold in just seven days of dieting?

The true culprit is living consistently in a caloric deficit and constantly burning fat for energy. When we don't break this pattern our leptin declines. Our brain is begging us to feast, so the way to restore leptin back to normal is give our brain exactly what it wants. We feast!

Research supports my theory

The evidence has been proven in studies. Following a period of calorie restriction, participants were then given a 12-hour period of overeating. Researchers found that leptin rose by 40-50% over baseline during the final hours of overfeeding; the increase persisted until the next morning! Unfortunately, the researchers didn't test any further than the following morning to see how long the increase lasted. What we do know is that leptin can decline drastically in as little as seven days, and a 12-hour period of overeating spikes leptin levels back up.

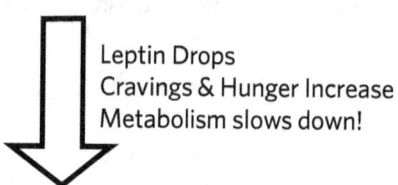
Leptin Drops
Cravings & Hunger Increase
Metabolism slows down!

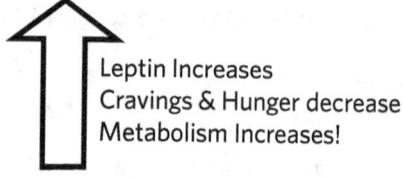
Leptin Increases
Cravings & Hunger decrease
Metabolism Increases!

How do we increase leptin levels?
We feast!

As you can see the answer to this problem is actually an obvious one. In order to avoid starvation mode, we need to follow days of calorie deficits with a day of calorie surplus. This is why in my book, *Spike Diet*, I tagged this glorious day as the Spike Day. Having a full day of a calorie surplus following six days of caloric deficits, spikes our leptin levels back up, and that in turn stops a dropping metabolism and decreases our food cravings.

Leptin Resistance

For most of us, when leptin levels are high, our brain has been signaled that we don't need to eat. Our cravings are gone and we are satisfied. Research then found a strange issue with some obese patients; their leptin levels were always high but yet they were still hungry. They found that leptin is similar to insulin in that if it is constantly high from years of overeating, then our body becomes less responsive to it.

This is why with Spike Life we create a caloric deficit for six days. During those six days our leptin levels will slowly decline, and when we have our Spike Day it will respond exactly the way we want by spiking back up and reducing our food cravings.

Leptin summary:
- Leptin is the anti-starvation hormone
- Leptin helps to regulate hunger and metabolism
- Leptin drops drastically after just seven days of calorie restriction
- When leptin is low we feel more hungry and our metabolism can slow
- Leptin spikes up after just a 12-hour period of overeating

Spike Life

- ▶ When leptin is balanced, hunger is avoided and metabolism is normal
- ▶ Spike Life maximizes the effects of leptin by spiking it up after it declines

CHAPTER 7

SPIKE DAYS

"Spiking works biochemically and psychologically by recharging your metabolism through hormone manipulation, as well as keeping you motivated to continue perusing your fitness goals. After a Spike Day, the process works by keeping you satisfied and crushing hunger cravings through the following week."—Dr. Christopher Balgobin, MD

Chapter 7 is about the amazing Spike Day. This one day plays a role in fixing several issues people face when trying to lose weight. It's the reason I was able to lose 100 pounds and maintain it. Get ready to spike your metabolism!

WHAT IS SPIKE DAY?

Conventional diets fail not because of some secret evil force trying to keep me or you fat, it's just our body's way of ensuring our survival. Our brain can do extraordinary things when pushed into a corner and this is no different. When we consistently restrict our calories, starvation mode will inevitably kick in, our metabolism will decline, and our fat-burning capabilities will slow to a halt.

One of the early signs of starvation mode is hunger and extreme food cravings. Our brain is pleading with us to feast, and at the same time we are begging our brain to let us lose weight. I say we give our brain what it wants and it will give us what we want. So we feast! A Spike Day is eating a surplus of calories for one day a week. Our brain is satisfied and in return our leptin levels spike back up, our metabolism spikes back up, our cravings go away, and mentally we get a break from diet foods and splurge on anything that was making us feel deprived. Everyone wins with a Spike Day.

Spiking is not cheating!

The general concept of overeating for a day has been used for many years by low-carb dieters and bodybuilders. They are often called "cheat-days" or carb re-feeds. The Spike Day is actually far from cheating. It's more beneficial than just reloading glycogen or giving your willpower a break. "Cheating" is a negative term, and the term "spiking" reminds us of the positive benefits. Not only does this satisfy our cravings, it also acts as a "reset" button for our diet. Like I said before, Spike Life is a series of six-day diets. You do not have to be overwhelmed with sticking to a diet and depriving yourself of your favorite foods for months and months. Instead, you are never more than a few days from enjoying your favorite meal. This is a powerful mental tool. During the week when you start to feel weak and cravings kick in, you just have to tell yourself you can wait a few more days and have it on your Spike Day. Spike Days will keep your metabolism from backfiring on you and give you control over your cravings. Starvation mode is the number one killer of diets with good intentions. With Spike Life, starvation mode will never get a chance to ruin your goals.

BENEFITS OF SPIKE DAYS

Spiking never allows our body adapt to a lower calorie intake

Our body is trying to stay in a state of homeostasis, and before our metabolism gets a chance to adapt, we have a Spike Day. It sends an *emphatic* message to our brain that we are not starving and it goes back to business as usual. Our metabolism stays strong and we go back to burning calories and body fat as usual.

Spike Days raise leptin and crushes food cravings after we spike

Spike Days increase our leptin levels, making us feel satisfied and destroying the cravings that were beginning to have an effect on us from calorie restriction.

Spike Days actually spike metabolism!

The calorie surplus from spiking causes the body to increase our basal metabolic rate (BMR) about 9% above baseline, and an even higher percentage is possible!

Spike Days improve your workouts

Spike Days allow us to restore our muscle glycogen, which is the stored glucose in our muscles used to fuel our workouts. Glycogen is often depleted when we diet. Restoring those calories by spiking provides enhanced strength and endurance for our upcoming workouts.

Spike Days give us a mental break

Who truly loves dieting? I sure don't. Spike Life gives you a break every week from dieting. That way, you are able to come back fresh and renewed; mentally, hormonally, and physically.

COMMON SPIKE DAY QUESTIONS

How many calories do I need to eat on Spike Day?

I define a Spike Day as 2X (BMR), or whatever you need to eat to ensure a *surplus* of calories. For most of us 2X (BMR) is a safe bet. You can find your Spike Day calorie goal in the calorie range chart in this book.

What kind of foods can you eat on Spike Day?

Another frequent question I get from clients is: "So I can eat a lot, but it's all healthy food right?" The answer is no, you can eat whatever you want. As far as the types of foods, I don't really have any food or meal restrictions, just a generous calorie goal to stick to.

I eat what I want and, specifically, what I crave. I usually have donuts, ice cream, pizza, cake, cookies, burgers, bratwurst, you name it. Whatever I've been craving, I have. I make a list during the week of foods I have been craving or wanting to try, and then on Spike Day I eat them, guilt-free!

If you don't want to eat a lot of junk food on your Spike Day, that's okay too. Just make sure you have a *surplus* of calories. If you want to eat extra calories from fruit, vegetables, and other healthy foods, go ahead.

I think it's fun to eat the "forbidden" foods while on a diet. It's redemption for all of those miserable years of dieting and food deprivation. It also makes for fun conversations. In the beginning, when I would see people that know me on my Spike Day, they would watch me in confusion while I ate donuts. Then they would say something like, "I thought you were on a diet." I would wink and say, "Yeah, I am. This is the new donut diet," and "You should try it." My joke doesn't work anymore but people definitely know when it's my Spike Day!

That's what I do, but it is not required that you eat junk food like me on your Spike Day. The only requirement is a surplus of calories.

Also, one cheat meal does not cut it. Studies show we need a *full day* of eating, or 12 hours, to make an impact on leptin and turn us back into fat-burning machines!

Am I supposed to exercise on Spike Day?

The answer is no, I do not recommend exercise on this day, as it defeats the purpose, and may hinder your chances of having a surplus of calories. You can exercise if you really want, but you may need to eat more calories.

Do I Really Take the day off from all things related to dieting?

Yes! You will refresh your body and your mind. This is a powerful benefit to living the Spike Life. Each week before your weight loss routine becomes dreadful. You get a one-day vacation from diet and exercise and it feels amazing!

I love my weekly break. I am thankful that I can eat these "forbidden" foods while losing weight, and not have a single guilty thought about it. By the end of the day, I am full, I am satisfied, and I am excited to get back to my healthy routine. The following day it's amazing how easy it is to go right back to a regular day. My cravings are wiped out and I'm motivated to see how much fat I will burn during the coming week.

Spike Day Summary

You don't have to eat junk foods like I do. If you're one of the few who doesn't care for those foods, just eat more of what you like, but it's imperative you get a *surplus* of calories. Again, you do not need to exercise on Spike Day.

Spike Day gives us a "reset" for our diet and we go back to normal, burning body fat for needed energy for another six days of having caloric deficits. With Spike Day, and varying our calorie intake daily, we keep our brain from lowering metabolism to a new energy balance point. Our hormones work on our side and we stay out of starvation mode. Spike Day allows you to become a continual *fat-burning machine*, decrease food cravings, and restore extremely important muscle glycogen. On top of that, we get to enjoy a day of eating any kind of food we want. Truly a win-win-win-win situation!

Spike Day

- ► Calorie goal is about 2 X (BMR)—Use chart in this book
- ► Drink extra water on Spike Day
- ► Take the day off from exercise
- ► You will temporarily gain 1-4 lbs of water weight from storing glycogen
- ► Enhances workouts for the following week and day after spiking
- ► Increases leptin levels
- ► Decreases hunger and cravings
- ► Mental break, a "day off" from all things diet related
- ► You're in control over your cravings and food choices
- ► Indulge in the foods you love, guilt-free
- ► You don't have to eat "junk food"
- ► Spikes metabolism and hormones for long-term weight loss
- ► May the Spike be with you!

CHAPTER 8

METABOLISM & SPIKE LIFE

The most important factor in losing weight is an obvious one, but one that is often overlooked, and that is your metabolism. We burn calories all day long, twenty four hours a day and seven days a week. Whether we are running on a treadmill or sitting on a couch and watching TV, our body is constantly using energy. In fact, most of the calories that we burn daily are from our resting metabolism. The problem with many of us who are overweight is that we have a low resting metabolism or basal metabolic rate (BMR). Your BMR is the number of calories you burn in a day *not* including strenuous activities like exercise. BMR is our *resting metabolism*, simply put, the calories we burn daily at rest. Unlike most diet programs that damage metabolism, Spike Life focuses on increasing resting metabolism through spiking and being active daily. Dieters are then able to lose more weight, and most importantly, keep it off after they reach their goal

Men typically have a much higher base metabolism because they have more muscle than women. It takes a higher amount of calories to maintain muscle, so the more muscle you have the more calories you burn daily.

Despite popular belief, metabolism does not shut down when we sleep. Many people are afraid to eat calories at night or before bed in fear that they will store those calories as fat since they are sleeping. In truth metabolism never stops, and our metabolism while sleeping is almost the same as it is while we are sitting at work or on a couch watching TV.

What is Metabolism?

For you and me, metabolism refers to the biochemical processes used to maintain life. These biochemical processes allow us to grow, reproduce, repair, and respond to our environment. Metabolism is responsible for our necessary functions, from our body moving, to our brain thinking, and our cells growing. In fact, there are thousands of metabolic functions that happen all at the same time. These functions are regulated by our hormones and our central nervous system.

There are two processes that make up what we call metabolism

- ▶ Catabolism—Creates energy
- ▶ Anabolism—Consumes energy

Catabolic Hormones—Break down tissue and create energy

Catabolism is the part of our metabolism that creates the energy needed to fuel everything we do. This includes breaking down the foods we eat into energy that our body can use, and creating energy from calories stored inside our body. Our body needs energy twenty four hours a day, and if we don't eat enough calories to provide that energy, our body uses catabolism to create it. Most of the time this stored energy comes from our fat cells. The catabolic hormones are:

- **Cortisol**—is known as the stress hormone. Cortisol is released in response to stress and anxiety. It increases blood pressure and blood sugar, and reduces the effectiveness of our immune system.
- **Glucagon**—is a hormone produced in our pancreas. It stimulates the breakdown of stored energy—glycogen and body fat—to get blood sugar levels to rise when there isn't enough sugar in our blood from the foods we consume. It also breaks down body fat for energy when our body needs calories.
- **Adrenalin**—causes the heartbeat to accelerate, strengthens the force of the heart's contraction, and opens up the bronchioles in the lung. This hormone is part of the "fight-or-flight" reaction animals and humans have in response to fear.

Anabolic Hormones—Consumes energy and builds tissue

Anabolism is the part of metabolism that uses energy to build, store, and create. Anabolic processes support the growth of new cells, the maintenance of body tissues, and the storage of energy for use in the future. Anabolism is the process used to build muscle but also store fat. The anabolic hormones are:

- **Growth hormone**—stimulates growth in our bodies and is extremely important for building muscle and burning body fat.
- **IGF1**—stimulates the production of protein. IGF1 is important for building and maintaining muscle.
- **Insulin**—a hormone produced in our pancreas. It regulates the level of sugar glucose in the blood. Our cells cannot utilize glucose without insulin. Insulin also drives amino acids and glycogen into our muscles.
- **Testosterone**—a male hormone that helps to strengthen muscles and bone mass.
- **Estrogen**—a female hormone also involved in strengthening bone mass.

Spike Life creates hormonal synergy

Hormones are extremely important to weight loss. In living the Spike Life we will have times of being both anabolic and catabolic. Our six days of caloric deficits will put us mainly in a catabolic state creating energy from tissue stored on our body. Spike Days are mainly anabolic, as our body will be able to build tissue from the extra calories we consumed spiking.

When we are healthy these two processes work together in perfect harmony like a beautiful symphony, but when we fail to respect the needs of our body it can be a symphony of mass destruction. We need to eat enough calories to allow our anabolic hormones to do their job building and maintaining muscle and restrict calories enough to allow our catabolic hormones to burn fat for energy. It's a complicated dance, but Spike Life is the master choreographer.

IMPORTANT SPIKE LIFE HORMONAL GOALS

HORMONE	GOAL	HOW TO MAXIMIZE THE BENEFITS
Insulin	Low	Keep blood sugar stable
Glucagon	High	Eat at a caloric deficit & keep blood sugar stable
Growth Hormone	High	Exercise, protein, and sleep 7-8 hours a night
Cortisol	Low	Live guilt-free and don't go to sleep hungry
Leptin	Low/High	6 days of calorie deficits and a Spike Day

METABOLISM AND SPIKE LIFE

Maximizing metabolism is the key to losing weight long term. Metabolism needs calories to function and we want a metabolism that requires lots of calories. Having a high metabolism gives you room for error with your eating; it's the reason why some people are able to eat whatever they want and not gain a pound. While they may have a calorie surplus, their BMR is high, so before excess calories get a chance to build up and store, their body burns it up for resting energy. For us "less fortunate," getting more active and eating the spike way is the only way to increase our metabolism without medical intervention. Constant dieting and exercise cause a hormonal imbalance and our metabolism is adversely affected. Spike Life breaks the mold of these conventional diets and uses a counterintuitive approach that actually makes sense and is also backed by scientific research.

What I've learned is that a diet should not starve you and, if it does, you will pay the price later as your metabolism will drop and all the weight you lost early on will come back with a vengeance.

Remember, our body has to metabolize each and every calorie we eat. Just like in physics, for each action there is an equal and opposite reaction. Eating causes metabolism to increase and not eating causes it to decrease. When we are consistently eating fewer and fewer calories, our metabolism quickly slows down simply because we are consuming fewer calories. Spiking is how we will keep our metabolism strong while we are losing weight.

Resting metabolism is responsible for burning the majority of our daily calories. As a weight loss bonus, our resting metabolism can get most of the energy it needs by burning body fat. While resting, the average person's metabolism burns about 70% of the calories it needs from stored body fat! This is the opposite of exercise, which uses mainly blood glucose and muscle glycogen for energy.

I am not saying we shouldn't exercise and just stay in bed all day. We do burn total calories at a much higher rate when we exercise than when we rest, and ultimately burning those extra calories creates a larger deficit that will allow us to lose more weight.

My point is that if 70% of our calories used for resting come from body fat, shouldn't we try to maximize our resting metabolism? Yes! Instead of letting our metabolism drop with a flat strict diet, we need to trick our body into maintaining and even spiking our metabolism to burn the most body fat!

Signs of an Unhealthy Metabolism

- ▶ Fatigue
- ▶ Insomnia
- ▶ Low morning body temperature
- ▶ Irritability
- ▶ Poor memory and concentration
- ▶ Heat and cold intolerance
- ▶ Weight gain

One of the issues with weight loss is that calorie restriction and cardio exercise can have a negative impact on metabolism. This is why maintaining weight loss is extremely difficult and many "lifelong dieters" find it more and more difficult to lose weight. Having a poor metabolism backs you into a corner where you are forced to exercise more and more and eat less and less to continue losing weight. This will not be the issue with Spike Life, because we make maximizing metabolism a priority.

How Spike Life Increases Metabolism

- ▶ Spike Day
- ▶ High protein meals
- ▶ High fiber meals
- ▶ Resistance training to build muscle
- ▶ Becoming more active, aim for 10,000 steps daily
- ▶ Eat a balanced diet

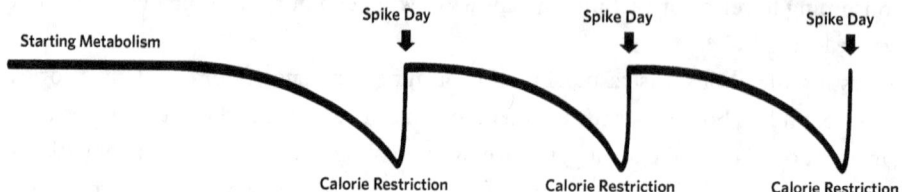

Calorie restriction causes our metabolism to decline and Spike Days spike it back up!

"CALORIES OUT"
Metabolism + Physical Activity + TEF

Calories Expended = BMR + Physical Activity + TEF

- ▶ BMR—Base Metabolism
- ▶ TDEE—Total Daily Energy Expenditure
- ▶ NEAT—Non-Exercise Activity Thermogenesis

BMR CHART

MEN WEIGHT	BMR	WOMEN WEIGHT	BMR
170lbs	1900	120lbs	1300
180lbs	1950	130lbs	1350
190lbs	2000	140lbs	1400
200lbs	2050	150lbs	1450
210lbs	2100	160lbs	1500
220lbs	2150	170lbs	1550
230lbs	2200	180lbs	1600
240lbs	2250	190lbs	1650
250lbs	2300	200lbs	1700
260lbs	2350	210lbs	1725
270lbs	2400	220lbs	1750
280lbs	2450	230lbs	1800
290lbs	2500	240lbs	1825
300lbs	2550	250lbs	1850
310lbs	2600	260lbs	1900
320bs	2650	270lbs	1925
330lbs	2700	280lbs	1950
340lbs	2750	290lbs	2000
350+lbs	2800	300+lbs	2050

Men have a higher BMR than women at the same weight because they typically have more pounds of lean body mass, which increases resting metabolism.

This is an easy to use but simplified BMR chart that is a good estimate of how many calories you burn daily just through your resting metabolism. The chart is based only on individual weight and sex. You can find a more complex and accurate BMR calculator online at spikelifebook.com

SPIKE LIFE DAILY CALORIE RANGES

Now that you know what BMR and metabolism is, it's time to find how many calories you should consume to lose weight with the Spike Life. Spike Life has a daily calorie range instead of a goal. This way you can eat more or less depending upon your hunger. You can choose to eat more with slower weight loss or less for quicker weight loss. I recommend eating more despite slower weight loss when you feel you need to. Feeling hungry makes us miserable and that will lead to quitting down the road.

SPIKE LIFE CALORIE TARGETS

MEN			WOMEN		
Body Weight	Calorie Range	Spike day Calories	Body Weight	Calorie Range	Spike day Calories
170lbs	1400-1900	3800	20lbs	1200-1300	2600
180lbs	1440-1950	3900	130lbs	1200-1350	2700
190lbs	1500-2000	4000	140lbs	1200-1400	2800
200lbs	1550-2050	4100	150lbs	1200-1450	2900
210lbs	1600-2100	4200	160lbs	1200-1500	3000
220lbs	1650-2150	4300	170lbs	1200-1550	3100
230lbs	1700-2200	4400	180lbs	1200-1600	3200
240lbs	1750-2250	4500	190lbs	1200-1650	3300
250lbs	1800-2300	4600	200lbs	1200-1700	3400
260lbs	1850-2350	4700	210lbs	1225-1725	3500
270lbs	1900-2400	4800	220lbs	1250-1750	3500
280lbs	1950-2450	4900	230lbs	1300-1800	3500
290lbs	2000-2500	5000	240lbs	1325-1825	3500
300lbs	2050-2550	5000	250lbs	1350-1850	3500
310lbs	2100-2600	5000	260lbs	1400-1900	3500
320bs	2150-2650	5000	270lbs	1425-1925	3500
330lbs	2200-2700	5000	280lbs	1450-1950	3500
340lbs	2250-2750	5000	290lbs	1500-2000	3500
62350+lbs	2300-2800	5000	300+lbs	1550-2050	3500

Spike Day

I cap men at 5,000 calories and women at 3,500 calories. Muscle mass, and not just overall weight, has the largest impact on our metabolism, so putting a cap on Spike Day calories still causes the caloric surplus we need to spike metabolism.

TOTAL DAILY ENERGY EXPENDITURE

TDEE is short for Total Daily Energy Expenditure. TDEE is a formula to estimate how many total calories we are burning daily from our base metabolism and our activity level, including exercise. I use TDEE to predict how much weight one could expect to lose with this weight loss plan. You can predict your weight loss by finding your TDEE and comparing that to your daily calorie goal. This is how we calculate calories in versus calories out.

To find your TDEE, simply multiply your BMR from the chart in this chapter by the activity multiplier below.

Total Daily Energy Expenditure (TDEE) = (BMR) X (Activity Multiplier)

Activity Multipliers

Sedentary = BMR x 1.2 (little or no exercise or activity)
Lightly active = BMR x 1.375 (exercise and activity 1-3 days/wk.)
Moderately active = BMR x 1.55 (exercise and activity 3-5 days/wk.)
Very active = BMR x 1.725 (exercise and activity 6-7 days/wk.)
Extremely active = BMR x 1.9 (daily exercise or physical job)
Calorie Surplus for Spike Day = BMR x 2

EXAMPLE:

Let's say Luke has a BMR of 2,000. He exercises 4 days a week and he's active daily, reaching his NEAT goal of 10,000 steps a day.

Luke's activity multiplier would be "Moderately Active" (BMR) X 1.55

2,000 X 1.55= Luke burns an average 3,100 calories a day or 21,700 calories a week.

This doesn't mean Luke burns 3,100 calories every single day. He will burn more on exercise days and less on non-exercise days, but 3,100 is his average calories burned a day per week for energy expenditure.

TDEE is much easier to track than trying to estimate and add up all of your calories burned through activities and exercise.

CALCULATE YOUR TDEE

Your TDEE = _____ x _____ = _____
                          BMR   *Activity Multiplier*

Weekly calories burned=_____ x 7 = _____
                                      TDEE

NON EXERCISE ACTIVITY (NEAT)

When most people want to lose weight they think of aerobics. They assume that by sweating an hour day by doing "cardio," they will burn fat and become lean. It's a very reasonable assumption, but new research has shown that exercise alone just doesn't do the trick. In fact, there is a more efficient way to increase your calorie output and maximize fat burning and it's not even exercise. It's called *non-exercise activity thermogenesis* or NEAT for short. NEAT is about all of the active movements our body makes that aren't considered traditional exercise. NEAT includes walking, fidgeting, standing, pacing, and things as simple as tapping your fingers. Researchers at the Mayo Clinic discovered that the reason that some people just seem to burn off excess calories versus those of us that just get fatter, was that the "thin" people had an increase NEAT after eating. Eating excess calories caused the lean group to just be more active. Obese people don't incorporate NEAT the same way.

The easiest ways to monitor NEAT is by wearing a pedometer. I recommend a goal of 10,000 steps a day. Walking 10,000 steps can burn an extra 500 calories daily or around 50 pounds of fat in a year! 10,000 steps are equal to about five miles of walking. You can choose to take one long walk a day or it may be easier to break that number up throughout the whole day.

Here are some simple ideas to incorporate 10,000 steps into your daily routine.

- ▶ Take a thirty minute walk after dinner
- ▶ Use the stairs instead of the elevator
- ▶ Walk the dog
- ▶ At stores, park in the back end of the parking lot
- ▶ Walk to the store
- ▶ Get up to change the channel
- ▶ Shop at malls or outdoor outlet malls
- ▶ Plan a neighborhood walking group

- ▶ Walk over to visit a neighbor
- ▶ Get outside to walk around the garden or do a little weeding
- ▶ Play games with your kids
- ▶ Play active video games, like dance or sport games
- ▶ Walk on a treadmill while you watch TV
- ▶ Jump on a mini-trampoline and listen to your favorite music
- ▶ At work, get up off your chair and walk around during breaks
- ▶ Make being active a daily priority

Don't be discouraged if you can't make the 10,000 steps goal early on. It may take some time getting used to it. Instead you can start small, like 4,000 steps and add 500 steps to your goal each week. The great thing about NEAT is every little bit counts and helps. The goal of Spike Life is living a manageable healthy lifestyle and the change doesn't always happen flawlessly overnight. It's more than OK to work up to the goals laid out in this book. I would rather you start small and gradually work your way to the goal than to have you get frustrated early and quit before this lifestyle can impact your life.

THERMIC EFFECT OF FOOD (TEF)

Part of metabolism is digesting and processing the foods we consume. It takes energy from our body to convert the calories from food to energy we can use. This process is called the Thermic Effect of Food or TEF for short. Every calorie we ingest has to be processed. This is why it's a myth that eating several small meals daily gives us a metabolic boost. It doesn't matter if we eat six small 300-calorie meals, or one large 1,800-calorie meal. Or if we eat a large breakfast or a large dinner, each one of those 1,800 calories is processed and gives us the same metabolic effect.

Different types of calories have different levels of TEF

Some calories give us a bigger metabolic boost than others; this is one reason why I say calories were not created equal. An easy way to understand this is food digestion. Foods that digest easily and quickly like processed carbohydrates and fats have a low TEF. While whole natural foods like vegetables and proteins take longer and require more energy from our body to digest.

This is another bonus of eating a high protein and fiber diet, and avoiding highly processed foods. In living the Spike Life, we want to consume foods that have a low calorie density and a high thermic effect.

Protein and Fiber have the highest TEF

Protein has the highest TEF, at around 30-33% and high fiber vegetables are second at 20%, while simple carbohydrates are just 6%, and fat is the lowest at 3%. The way this works is if we eat 100 protein calories, our body will burn about 30 calories just to process the protein into amino acids and utilize them. In contrast if we have 100 calories from dietary fat, it will burn 3 calories to utilize it. Hot spicy foods can also increase the thermic effect of food. Interestingly, alcohol also has a high TEF at 20%, but I wouldn't call it a good food choice.

High protein diet versus a low protein diet

TEF can really add up over time. Say, for example, we have two identical people eating the same caloric goal. One consumes 40 grams of protein daily, *low protein* (LP). The other consumes 140 grams of protein daily, *high protein* (HP).

The (HP) diet person will burn an extra 100 calories daily more than the (LP) person by simply consuming a higher percentage of protein calories. Over a year that difference is more than ten pounds of fat. Remember, these are identical people with the same calorie goal, but the high protein diet burns more calories!

The Average American Diet versus the Spike Life Plan

The average American diet produces an overall thermic effect of about 10%. If one consumes 2,000 calories, they will burn 200 calories in the process. With Spike Life we eat a high protein and high fiber diet producing an average thermic effect of 14%. With the same 2,000 calories, we burn 280 calories in the process. 80 calories may not seem like very much, but over a year, it's 29,200 calories or an extra 8 lbs a year by simply eating a higher protein and fiber diet.

TEF proves each calorie was not created equal

- ▶ Protein 30-33%
- ▶ Fibrous Fruits and Vegetables 20%
- ▶ Carbohydrate 6%
- ▶ Dietary Fat 3%

Spices that can increase TEF

- ▶ Hot Peppers
- ▶ Cayenne Pepper
- ▶ Hot Sauces
- ▶ Cinnamon
- ▶ Garlic
- ▶ Ginger
- ▶ Mustards
- ▶ Parsley
- ▶ Celery Seed

PREDICTING FAT LOSS THROUGH CALORIE RANGES AND TDEE

I use TDEE to estimate how much weight one could expect to lose with the Spike Life plan. Remember, the average American diet provides a thermic effect of about 10%. Spike Life is high protein and fiber diet so it creates an average thermic effect of 14%. The types of calories we eat living the Spike Life burns more calories than the average American diet through TEF.

AN EXAMPLE OF SOMEONE WITH A BMR OF 2,000

TOTAL CALORIES EXPENDED = TDEE (BMR X ACTIVITY MULTIPLIER)

BMR	2,000 calories
X (Activity Multiplier)	1.55 (moderate)
TDEE	3,100 calories (2,000 x 1.55)
Calories Burned Daily	3,100
Calories Burned Weekly	21,700

TOTAL CALORIES CONSUMED:

Calorie Range	1,500–2,000 calories
Three "Low Days"	1,500 X 3(days) = 4,500
Three "High Days"	2,000 X 3(days) = 6,000
Spike Day	4,000 calories

TOTAL "CALORIES IN" VS. "CALORIES OUT" FOR THE WEEK:

Total "Calories In"	14,500 calories consumed weekly
Total "Calories Out"	18,975 calories burned weekly
Net Weekly Calorie Deficit	-7,200 calories (14,500—21,700)

TOTAL PROJECTED FAT LOSS:
7,200/3500 = 2.05 lbs of fat lost per week /106 per year
(One Pound of Fat equals 3,500 Calories)

AN EXAMPLE OF SOMEONE WITH A BMR OF 1,500	
TOTAL CALORIES EXPENDED = TDEE (BMR X ACTIVITY MULTIPLIER)	
BMR	1,500 calories
X (Activity Multiplier)	1.75 (very active)
TDEE	2,625 calories (1,500 x 1.75)
Calories Burned Daily	2,625
Calories Burned Weekly	18,975
TOTAL CALORIES CONSUMED:	
Calorie Range	*1,200–1,500 calories*
Three "Low Days"	1,200 X 3(days) = 3,600
Three "High Days"	1,500 X 3(days) = 4,500
Spike Day	3,000 calories
TOTAL "CALORIES IN" VS. "CALORIES OUT" FOR THE WEEK:	
Total "Calories In"	11,100 calories consumed weekly
Total "Calories Out"	18,975 calories burned weekly
Net Weekly Calorie Deficit	-7,875 calories (11,100—18,975)

TOTAL PROJECTED FAT LOSS:
7,875 / 3500= 2.25 lbs fat loss per week/ 140lbs year
(One Pound of Fat equals 3,500 Calories)

You can see by these examples that the more active you are, the more weight you can expect to lose. I feel the safe range for fat loss is 1-3 lbs per week. If we try to lose more we risk losing lean body mass in the process, which will ultimately lower our metabolism. These are ideal examples of people losing weight living the Spike Life. The people in these examples could choose to consume more calories and have 6 "high days" and they will still lose 1-2 lbs per week. This is where you have a choice and control over your weight loss.

PREDICT YOUR WEEKLY FAT LOSS WORKSHEET
Use the charts in this chapter and the examples above

TOTAL CALORIES EXPENDED = TDEE (BMR X ACTIVITY MULTIPLIER)

BMR	
X (Activity Multiplier)	
TDEE	
Calories Burned Daily	
Calories Burned Weekly	

TOTAL CALORIES CONSUMED:

Calorie Range (from chart)	calories
Three "Low Days"	X 3(days) =
Three "High Days"	X 3(days) =
Spike Day	calories

TOTAL "CALORIES IN" VS. "CALORIES OUT" FOR THE WEEK:

Total "Calories In"	calories consumed weekly
Total "Calories Out"	calories burned weekly
Net Weekly Calorie Deficit	calories

TOTAL PROJECTED FAT LOSS:

_____ /3500= _____ lbs fat loss per week/ _____ lbs year
(One Pound of Fat equals 3,500 Calories)

If you're not satisfied with your predicted weight loss, you can have more days in the lower range of your calorie goals and exercise more often. Remember, Spike Life is about living a manageable healthy lifestyle where you can lose weight and maintain your weight loss. This is not a "crash diet" designed to lose a bunch of weight up front and put you in a position where it's impossible to maintain it. We are stopping the insanity and losing weight in a fun and healthy way.

ENERGY BALANCE SUMMARY
Energy Balance= Calories consumed versus calories expended

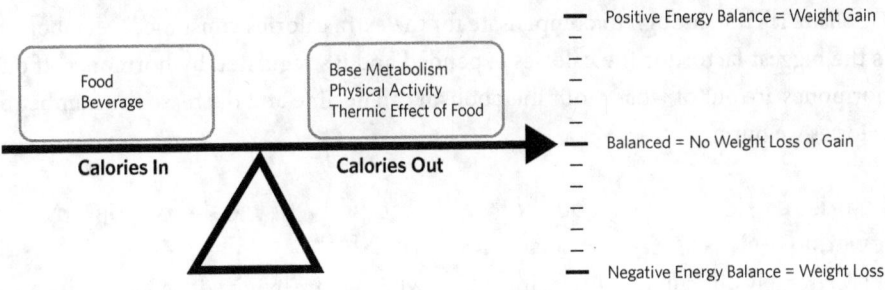

The Ultimate Battle for Weight Loss

It is very true that we gain and lose weight determined by the Law of Thermodynamics. If we expend more energy than we consume, we burn stored energy to make of the deficit and lose weight. When we consume a surplus of calories, our body stores the excess calories and we gain weight. Now you understand that body fat isn't the only way we store energy. Glycogen is what I call a dieter's best friend since it acts as the buffer between excess calories and body fat. Also, by manipulating our daily caloric intake, we can maximize the effectiveness of glycogen and get the benefits of extraordinary workouts at the same time we are losing weight.

If losing weight is as simple as calories in vs. calories out, then why is it not that easy!?

The truth is that losing weight never was as simple as calories in versus calories out, even though that was engrained in my head by my doctors and trainers in the past. I believed in the Law of Thermodynamics but I knew there had to be more to it.

There were many times that I thought should be a caloric deficit based on the numbers, but yet I wasn't losing weight. My trainer would accuse me of lying or manipulating my numbers, but I wasn't. I was honest with myself and him, but it still wasn't working.

I still believe the Law of Thermodynamics is unbreakable but now know it can be bent. There are numerous variables that can have an adverse effect on our energy balance but the two main ones relate to the types and amounts of calories we consume.

The amounts of calories and the types of calories we consume directly influence the number of calories we expend.

For example, if we consume 1,000 calories, our body has to metabolize 1,000 calories through our metabolism. Now if we consume 5,000 calories, our body has to metabolize 5,000 calories, causing a greater increase in metabolism than consuming 1,000 calories did. I'm not telling you to always eat more, because while it does increase metabolism, it's not enough to compensate for the extra calories consumed. Metabolism is the biggest factor for the calories expended and it's regulated by hormones. If our hormones are out of whack, our metabolism can decline and decrease the number of calories we burn.

Calorie restriction makes our body adapt to find a new balance point by lowering our resting metabolism.

It is extremely difficult to burn fat for energy when we are living with a slower metabolism. Little did I know in the past that my diet and my constant exercise was making me become like a hamster on a wheel; no matter how hard I tried, I was getting nowhere. With Spike Life we can vary our caloric intake daily, and with a weekly Spike Day we never let our body adapt to fewer calories.

PART II

HUNGER AND CRAVINGS

Introduction
Hunger & Cravings on a Diet

Chapter 9
Physical Hunger

Chapter 10
Mental & Emotional Cravings

Key Terms:

Satiety—Satiety is the feeling of being full and satisfied from food.

VLCD—Very Low Calorie Diet, usually 500–800 calories a day.

Ghrelin—Hormone that makes you feel hungry.

Empty Calories—Types of foods that are calorie dense, meaning there are many calories with little nutritional benefit.

Nutrient Dense—These foods provide us plenty of nutritional needs with fewer calories.

INTRODUCTION

HUNGER AND CRAVINGS ON A DIET

Two of the biggest obstacles when trying to lose weight are cravings and hunger. We all have good intentions when we begin a healthy lifestyle, but our hunger and cravings have a strong hold on us. I love food, you probably love food. There's a reason that we are overweight to begin with. Unfortunately, these cravings don't simply go away because we ask them to. In my experience I've learned that we deal with both emotional and physical cravings while dieting. In creating the Spike Lifestyle I've come up with plans of action to defuse these situations before they happen and emergency plans to stop them from becoming disastrous. With Spike Life you should never have to deal with being hungry, and cravings will not be an issue, as you won't feel deprived. You will also see another benefit of Spike Days and how they have a positive physiological and mental effect on cravings and hunger.

The two main types of hunger that make losing weight difficult:

▶ Physical Hunger
▶ Emotional Cravings

Reasons why we have constant hunger and cravings while dieting:

▶ Calorie restriction
▶ Poor food choices (processed foods and calorie dense foods)
▶ Feeling deprived
▶ Hormonal changes
▶ Stress

CHAPTER 9

PHYSICAL HUNGER

Physical hunger is not something in our heads, and it doesn't involve willpower. It's hard to be successful losing weight when we are always hungry. Spike Life has a plan of action so that you can consume fewer calories and not feel physically hungry all day.

> *You are sitting in on a big office meeting; the room is in a dead silence. Everyone is waiting for the boss to finish up his talk so you can go to lunch. Then, at the most embarrassing of moments, you feel a twinge and your stomach growls to break the silence. Sound familiar?*

These awkward moments happen to all of us, especially when we are dieting. The truth is when this happens, you just need to eat. I have learned from experience that it is awfully difficult to stick to a healthy lifestyle if we are always hungry.

When I'm physically hungry my willpower fails, and I would eat just about anything offered to me, no matter the consequences. A big part of living the Spike Life is that we a have plan of action to avoid these situations. In those rare times that we do feel uncontrollable hunger, Spike Life has a plan to troubleshoot our cravings to keep us from falling off the deep end and binging on french fries and onion rings.

WHY ARE WE PHYSICALLY HUNGRY?

Reasons we may feel physically hungry

- ▶ Ghrelin
- ▶ Leptin
- ▶ Insufficient calories
- ▶ Poor meal choices

Ghrelin

Ghrelin is a hormone that tells us it's time to eat, literally. Research has shown that our brain adapts to the time of day we typically eat. This is one reason why people who skip breakfast are telling the truth when they say they are not hungry. It's important to know that if you are making changes to your diet that it might take some time for ghrelin to adjust to your new pattern. When ghrelin is high we are hungrier, and after we eat, ghrelin levels dip and we are satisfied. Research has shown that over time our baseline levels of ghrelin decrease when we restrict calories and lose weight. So in a sense, your hunger will decrease in due time.

The best way to keep your ghrelin low is to eat foods that have slow digestion like fiber and protein. Eating these types of foods will keep hunger away for hours.

> **!** SPIKE LIFE TIP
> Drinking water between meals can reduce ghrelin and hunger. For an even better effect add fiber powder to your water.

Leptin

You already know that leptin levels decline with caloric restriction. When leptin levels are low, our cravings increase. Spike Day spikes leptin back up so our cravings can leave us alone.

Insufficient calorie consumption

The obvious answer is that we are not eating enough calories. While it's kind of true, I would actually say it's probably the wrong answer. The best answer is we are consuming insufficient *types* of calories.

You can choose meals with the exact number of calories and be really hungry after one, and be satisfied for hours after the other. Calories are important but do not tell the full story.

For example, let's compare two 500-calorie meals

Meal #1—500 Calories
► Macaroni and cheese
► Bag of chips
► Pop

Meal #2—500 Calories
► Grilled chicken breast
► Steamed broccoli with cheese
► Milk

Now let me ask you, do you think there's a chance that Meal #2 will make you feel full longer than Meal #1? They are both 500 calories.

If you answered yes, that Meal #2 will make you feel full longer, then you are correct. It also shows us that hunger isn't just caused by the amount of calories we consume. This is extremely important because weight loss is determined by the Law of Thermodynamics: calories in versus calories out. If we can lower the amount of calories we consume we will lose more weight. However, remember in the Spike Life that every calorie was NOT created equal.

Some calories we consume are quickly processed and spend very little time in digestion. Those calories are quickly burned for energy and we are hungry again soon after. These foods are called empty calories or calorie dense.

Calorie Dense Foods Keep Us Hungry
I'm sure you have heard the expression "empty calories"; these are foods that are highly processed and lack any nutritional benefit to our bodies.

Examples of Empty Calories
- Candy
- Chips
- Cookies
- Crackers
- White bread
- Alcohol
- Soda Pop
- Juice (it has some vitamins, but the amount is not worth the calorie content)
- Foods deep fried in trans fats
- Many processed foods

Consuming too many of our calories from "empty calories" leads to cravings and hunger, and us going over our daily calorie range.

If we are not getting the nutrients we need, our brain will cause us to be hungry and crave more food in an effort to get us to eat more.

It happens often with pregnant women and their strange cravings. They can come directly from a lack of nutrients. When our body senses a deficiency of vital nutrients, our cravings go up in an effort to satisfy our needs. If your goal is to lose weight, this is why empty calories should be avoided during our non-Spike Days. Otherwise those empty calories will be burned for energy instead of stored body fat, and even worse, they won't do anything to impede our hunger and cravings. People who choose to eat meals full of empty calories tend to overeat simply because they are always hungry.

An important factor to avoiding physical hunger is to get the nutrients we need. While empty calories are processed quickly and make us hungry quicker, other calories take more time and more energy to process and digest. These calories keep us full longer so we can stretch out the time longer between meals.

By having a breakfast of eggs, Canadian bacon, and fruit—instead of a bowl of cereal and a processed granola bar—you will have a much better chance stretching out the time to your next meal. Then you will be able to avoid those embarrassing moments of a loud stomach growl while at work. More importantly, you can avoid those times when you are extremely hungry and presented with one of my biggest vices: free food! This is, and will always be, one of my biggest obstacles. But if I can keep my hunger to a minimum, I am able to keep my willpower and self-control at a maximum.

Nutrient Dense Foods

When choosing our daily menu, we need to focus on foods that are nutrient dense or what I call "Spike Life Priority Foods." This way, we will accomplish our fitness goals without the agony of constant physical hunger. With Spike Life you can eat a variety of different foods, but nutrient dense foods are essential.

Nutrient dense foods are the direct opposites of calorie dense foods. For me, visually, it's easiest to explain by comparing 1,000 calories of ice cream to 1,000 calories of broccoli. 1,000 calories of ice cream is about 4 cups; it will actually fit in a large bowl, while you would need to eat about 33 cups of broccoli to get 1,000 calories. Can you see how, even though they have an equal amount of calories, this comparison is far from being equal? I could eat, and I have eaten 1,000-plus calories of ice cream, and a few minutes later went back for more. I don't think it's physically possible to eat 1,000 calories of broccoli, and if I did, I'd be full for hours! These high volume foods take up a lot more space in your stomach, and process much slower than empty calorie foods.

The fact is we need to eat fewer calories than we burn to lose weight. This makes it important to choose foods that provide us a high level satiety. Making good food choices for meals helps tremendously to avoid hunger.

For example:

Someone with a BMR of 2,000 could be satisfied on just 1,500 calories a day by choosing *nutrient dense* foods, but struggle with hunger if they eat 2,500 calories if their meals are comprised of mainly *empty calories*.

Nutrient Dense Foods
- ▶ Poultry
- ▶ Lean Grass-Fed Meat
- ▶ Fish
- ▶ High Fiber Vegetables
- ▶ Potatoes
- ▶ Fruit
- ▶ High Fiber Whole Grains

- Eggs
- Starchy Vegetables
- Legumes
- Nuts
- Greek Yogurt
- Beef Jerky
- Reduced-Fat Cheese Sticks

SPIKE LIFE TIP

I often choose reduced-fat options for foods because they generally have less overall calories than the full-fat version. However, some food manufactures replace the fat with sugar or HFCS; I avoid these options and choose the regular full-fat version. This is when reading food labels is very important. If the reduced-fat version has the same number of calories than the original, then it usually has added calories from sugar. Just remember a food labeled "low-fat" doesn't mean it's healthy.

Each calorie was not created equal

Remember the quality of a calorie is just as important as the quantity when it comes to hunger. If the goal is weight loss, getting essential dietary needs is the most important factor when planning meals. We can't win our case in the Law of Thermodynamics if we are deficient in vitamins, minerals, amino acids, essential fatty acids, and fiber. Our body will not operate at peak efficiency if it's lacking those necessary nutrients.

If you choose the right foods, you can give your body the nutrients it needs while in a caloric deficit. A caloric deficit is necessary for weight loss and we have plenty of stored energy (calories) trapped inside our body, ready to be released, when energy is needed.

SPIKE LIFE TIP

High protein and fiber foods provide a very high level of satiety. These foods need to become the staples of our diet.

FOOD FULLNESS GRADES

Foods that have a high ratio of fiber and protein make us feel fuller per calorie than foods that are low in fiber and protein. While losing weight ultimately comes down to just calories in versus out, it can be hard to stick to a lower calorie goal if we are always hungry. Spike Life has a list of common foods graded A+ to F for their fullness per calorie. Since dietary fats have the highest amount of calories per gram, fats and oils are generally graded lower on the fullness scale.

FOODS GRADED ON FULLNESS PER CALORIE

A+	A	B+	B
Bean sprouts	Oranges	Popcorn	Quinoa
Watermelon	Fish, broiled	Baked potato	Brown rice
Grapefruit	Grilled chicken	Greek yogurt	Low fat yogurt
Carrots	Apples	Banana	Fiber bars
Broccoli	Sirloin steak	High fiber Cereal	Rolled oats

C+	C	D+	D
Spaghetti	Pizza	Ice cream	Candy Bar
Macaroni & Cheese	White Rice	White bread	Honey
Cereal & Milk	Peanuts	Raisins	

F
Sugar
Potato chips
Snack cakes
Butter
Soda
Juice
Oils

CHAPTER 10

MENTAL & EMOTION CRAVINGS

"There is a charm about the forbidden that makes it unspeakably desirable."
—Mark Twain

There's the saying, "we want what we can't have." This is very true when we are dieting. Most of us are overweight because we love food. This love doesn't simply go away because we want to lose weight and be fit. As much as we may want to give up certain foods, our connections are too strong and it's nearly impossible to say goodbye forever.

The reason we love "junk food"

Calorie dense foods—"junk food"—are the perfect drug for our brain. There's a reason why we are strongly connected to foods like cookies, pizza, and ice cream. There's a reason why they taste so darn good. Our brain likes easy energy, the kinds of foods that require very little of our own energy to metabolize, yet supply our body with plenty of energy from calories. Calorie dense foods are like premium fuel for our body and our brain wants us to consume them. We are drawn to high calorie, sweet foods. We are drawn to fatty foods, too; doesn't adding oil or butter to foods make them taste even better? Taste is controlled by our brain; if it wanted us to eat broccoli all day, then it would taste like chocolate. It's important to understand that cravings have very little to do with willpower and a lot to do with the way we are hardwired. We need to quit putting pressure on ourselves to be perfect with our food decisions and quit feeling guilty when we're not perfect. Instead, we need to understand why we struggle with cravings, and devise an action plan to deal with them before they become an issue.

Emotional cravings happen even when we are not physically hungry, and if we can ignore them, sometimes they eventually go away. The problem is they always come back. This is emotional, it's "true love"; even when we let them go, they always return. I know these emotional cravings all too well, so while living the Spike Life, I created action plans to deal with the triggers to our emotional cravings.

ACTION PLANS TO CONTROL YOUR CRAVINGS

Things that can trigger our emotional cravings

- ▶ Aroma
- ▶ Habit
- ▶ Boredom

- ▶ Feeling sad
- ▶ Deprivation
- ▶ Celebration

Food Aroma

The aroma of my favorite foods gets me all the time. When I'm grocery shopping and walk by the bakery section where they are making fresh donuts, or driving past fast food restaurants when I can literally smell the burgers on the grill, my mouth waters and my cravings are triggered.

Plan of action: I always carry mints or mint gum with me. All it takes is a second of strength to pop one in my mouth; doing so would ruin the taste of even the most delicious treat. At home I can brush my teeth for the same effect.

Habitual Eating

I've always been a habitual eater. I love eating food while I watch TV at night and I also like eating in the car. In the past I would stop for fast food often just because of habit. Over the years we have all created eating habits.

Plan of action: I know what truly matters is overall calories for the day, so I adjusted my daily meal plan by eating less calories early in the day to allow more calories at night. This way I can eat while I watch TV but still be within my calorie range. While driving I have the gum trick still, but I also keep healthy snacks like beef jerky in my car so I can eat without stopping for fast food.

Many gas stations sell beef jerky, protein bars, and ready to drink protein shakes now too. So if you do stop, you have healthy options.

If I do stop for fast food, most of the places sell some sort of grilled chicken. The trick to eating fewer calories at fast food restaurants is to order your meal without the extras like mayo, dressing, or cheese.

Since Spike Life allows for flexibility in your meal plans, you can customize your daily calories to fit with your most of your current eating habits.

Boredom

When I'm bored I find myself wanting to go to the refrigerator or pantry to find something to do, and technically, eating is doing something. Usually when we are bored we are also not happy, and emotionally we know food can make us happy.

Plan of action: Go ahead and grab some food, but instead of reaching for a quick snack, prepare a healthy meal or snack for later. I have outstanding high protein recipes in this book that you can use for examples. End your boredom by experimenting with your own healthy recipes. That way you are busy, you can taste what you're making, and later when you are actually hungry you will have something good to eat. One of my favorite skills I learned during my personal weight loss journey was cooking healthy. I found ways to adapt some of my favorite unhealthy foods into healthy and delicious versions.

Sadness

This is a huge stereotype, but it's true; we are feeling terrible, so we grab a spoon and the box of ice cream out of the freezer and eat our sadness away. While we know that eating our sadness away only works temporarily and actually makes us feel worse when we're done, it doesn't stop us in the moment when immediate satisfaction is wanted.

Plan of action: Write down all of the things not food related that make you happy. Call them your "Happy List" and do this now, when you are happy and motivated. Then the next time you want to curl up with a pint of ice cream, grab your "Happy List" and start doing the things that make you happy.

My Happy List

- ▶ Play with my boys
- ▶ Listen to music
- ▶ Write
- ▶ Play video games
- ▶ Talk to friends and family
- ▶ Exercise
- ▶ Watch a funny movie
- ▶ Look at my weight loss progress pictures
- ▶ Thank God for all of the good things in my life
- ▶ Visualize my dream life
- ▶ Volunteer to help someone

Deprivation

We want things more when we can't have them, and this is very true for diets. Besides not working, diets make us miserable because we give up things that we love for what we hope will be a healthier and thinner body. Feeling deprived is a huge deal and I think the #1 reason people don't stick to a diet. I know some say that we are food addicts, and if we go quit cold turkey, eventually we will stop craving those foods. I have personal experience with giving up my favorite foods. For almost two years I didn't eat pizza, ice cream, or most junk foods because I was sure those foods were the reason I was overweight. During that time my love and cravings never went away. Feeling deprived was just as awful as being overweight. Eventually I quit that nonsense, but I was in such a bad place mentally that once I began eating them again, I couldn't stop. I was splurging daily and I gained weight back as fast as I lost.

Plan of action: Unlike most diets, you will not feel deprived with Spike Life. You are always within days of your next Spike Day when you can eat anything you desire.

Celebration

Let's say you just got a huge job promotion and your boss wants to take you out to celebrate. Food is always connected to celebrating, whether it's a birthday, holiday, or just amazing news.

Plan of action: Enjoy and celebrate your great news! Yes, I mean it. Spike Life is about control and creating positive food connections. Many of us have negative connections to food, and celebrations are a positive connection. It's not a big deal if it's not your Spike Day. Going over on your calories one extra day a week once in a while is not going to harm your progress. Birthdays and holidays are always free *extra* Spike Days. Now, don't get carried away. I'm not talking about half-birthdays or Flag Day, but for big celebrations like Christmas. It doesn't matter what day it falls on, I'm definitely spiking. You can tone it down a bit and not do an all-out Spike, and instead have a Spike meal or throw in some non-healthy foods throughout the day if that makes you feel better. Or you could just move your once a week Spike Day to that day.

YOU "FELL OFF THE WAGON"

Let's be honest, this happens to the best of us. Even when we are not deprived and living the Spike Life, a craving may come out of nowhere and we give in. It may be pressure from someone we care about or a moment where we forgot who was in control.

The most important part of falling off is getting right back on. The best way to do this is to forgive your lapse of judgment and move on. Just forget about it! There is no room for guilt in Spike Life. This book is about living a fun and healthy life, and part of life is making mistakes. It happens to everyone, it happens to me. I know that guilt is far more damaging than extra calories. So I forgive and forget. I don't use this as an excuse to *fall off the wagon* whenever I want to. Instead, I use it as a learning experience of how and why I did it so that I can avoid doing it again in the future. I don't punish myself with extra cardio or excessively low calories the next day. I just get myself back on the right track and move forward.

When we live the Spike Life we are not as deprived as we are on most weight loss plans, so we are far less likely to fall. We are in control, and on our planned Spike Day, we safely jump off the wagon and enjoy our break, guilt-free. It's much easier to get back on the wagon the next day when you safely jump off. You avoid the injuries that can happen when you fall.

Potential diet sabotage situation or not: What should you do?

Your best friend is having a birthday party, and it happens to be mid-week and your Spike Day isn't until Saturday. You know there's going to be pizza, snacks, and of course, cake with ice cream. You are starting to feel anxiety over the occasion because you love parties and cake, but you have done so well with weight loss that you don't want to blow it. What are you going to do?

This situation happens to all of us when we are dieting, but with Spike Life you are no longer dieting, you are living a lifestyle.

What would I do?

I'm going to the party and I am going to eat what I want without remorse, guilt, or fear.

We have learned that what really matter is calories in versus calorie out. I would adjust my daily meals to allow myself the extra calories I need to eat what I want and enjoy the party. If I have time, I may fit in an extra workout before the party to increase my calorie output, and I would definitely eat fewer calories before the party. I make sure the calories I consume before are the best of the best. I eat lots of fiber and protein, and save my carbohydrate and fat calories for the pizza and cake. To keep myself from overeating, I also would eat a high protein and fiber snack or meal just before the party. That way I would be much more likely to enjoy the party foods in moderation. I would also use one of my favorite tips, and bring mint gum to have after I eat. Mint ruins the flavor of food and this will prevent me from hovering around the food table and munching the entire night.

Hunger & Cravings Summary

▶ The longer it takes food to digest, the longer we feel full.
▶ Natural foods high in fiber and protein provide the most fullness.
▶ Processed foods are digested very quickly and leave us hungry.
▶ Everyone who is trying to lose weight deals with cravings and hunger.
▶ If you "fall off the wagon," get right back on and let go of your guilt.
▶ Refer to the section on troubleshooting if you find yourself struggling.

PART IV

CALORIES

Key Terms:

Blood Glucose or Blood Sugar—The sugar our body makes from food. It is carried in our bloodstream to provide energy to all of our cells.

Hypoglycemia—When you blood sugar crashes and you feel lethargic, having almost flu-like symptoms. When blood sugar returns to normal, you feel better.

Insulin Resistance—This is when our body does not react to insulin like it should, and it can no longer regulate blood sugar.

Processed Food—These are foods that have been altered from their natural state.

INTRODUCTION

CALORIES

From vegetables to donuts, all food has calories. The truth is weight loss is a product of consuming fewer calories than we expend. You could lose weight if you only ate donuts, and you could potentially gain weight if you only ate vegetables, although it would have to be a lot of vegetables.

The Law of Thermodynamics

The Law of Thermodynamics is the "black and white" answer to weight loss. It's a mathematical equation that states: "Calories In" vs. "Calories Out" = Weight Loss or Weight Gain.

However, we don't live in a "black and white" world, and losing weight has never been as simple as eating less and exercising more.

The Shades of Gray

The foods that we choose to eat are more than just calories. They can have positive or negative effects on our hormones, hunger, and metabolism. Spike Life promotes eating the types of food that promote positive changes. These are natural foods that are high in protein, fiber, and essential fats. We want to limit highly processed foods, including sugars, white starches, and hydrogenated fats.

You will learn in this chapter that different types of calories make you fuller than others, and they can also provide a larger boost to your metabolism. Other foods may be very high in calories but provide very few nutritional benefits and leave you hungry and ready to eat again soon after.

Unhealthy Processed Foods

Processed foods have been altered from their natural state for food preservation or convenience. This includes canning, freezing, refrigeration, dehydration, and sterilization. When I talk about *avoiding processed foods* I am directly referring to the ones that add high fructose corn syrup and trans fats. These additives are cheap for manufacturing and they help lengthen the shelf life of food, along with adding calories. For us, these additives have been shown to raise LDL cholesterol, blood sugar, and mess with our hormones. Check labels and avoid foods that contain high fructose corn syrup (corn sugar) and hydrogenated oils (trans fats). Technically, frozen vegetables and fruits are processed foods, but I have them frequently because freezing them locks in their vitamins and minerals at the peak of freshness.

IMPORTANT SPIKE LIFE CALORIE PRINCIPLES

You know weight loss is determined by calories in versus calories out. As long as you stick within your Spike Life calorie range, you will create a weekly caloric deficit and lose weight despite the types of food you choose to eat. However, I'm telling you from experience that it is extremely difficult to stick to eating fewer calories when you make less than ideal food choices. By following the Spike Life Principles for calories and meal planning, you will have a much easier time consuming fewer calories. By choosing the right types of foods, you will feel less hungry, keep your blood sugar stable, and as an added bonus, you will boost your metabolism with a greater thermic effect of food (TEF).

Spike Life Calorie Principles
- ▶ Choose natural options for food
- ▶ Prioritize protein and fiber
- ▶ 7–10g of protein per 100 calories
- ▶ 7–10g of carbohydrates per 100 calories
- ▶ 3–4g of natural fats per 100 calories
- ▶ 2–3g of fiber per 100 calories
- ▶ Avoid highly processed foods

Spike Life Formula for Success
- ▶ Find your calorie range
- ▶ 34% Proteins—33% Carbohydrates—33% Fats
- ▶ 30–50 grams of Fiber
- ▶ Use the Spike Life Food Pyramid of for Meal Planning

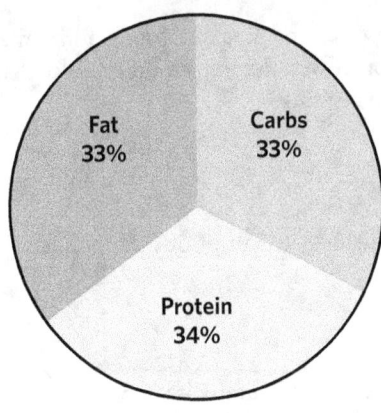

Spike Life Food Pyramid

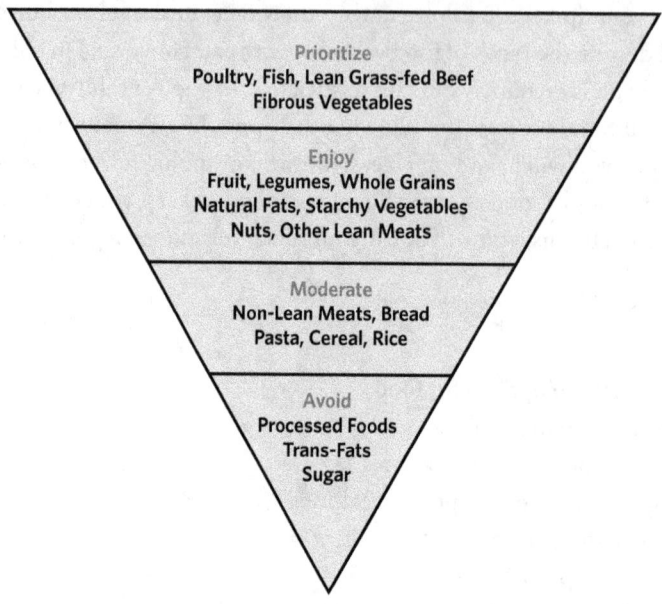

Prioritize—Every Meal

These are the foods we want to include in every meal. Priority foods help us stabilize blood sugar, boost metabolism, and provide us with hours of satiety.

> **!** SPIKE LIFE TIP
>
> When eating *Avoid* and *Moderate* foods, add some *Priority* foods to the meal to slow digestion, lessen the impact on our blood sugar, and reduce the corresponding insulin response.

Enjoy—Half of Daily Meals

These foods we should include in half of our daily meals. They are healthy but are generally higher in calories.

Enjoy Foods:

Fruit, Legumes, Whole Grains, Natural Fats, Starchy Vegetables, Nuts, Other Lean Meats

Moderate—One or Two Daily Meals

These foods we could include in one or two of our daily meals. They are high in calories without the additional nutritional benefits that are in the *Priority* and *Enjoy* foods.

Moderate Foods:
Non-Lean Meats, Bread, Pasta, Cereal, Rice

Avoid—Limit to Spike Day
These foods should be kept at a minimum. I save them for my Spike Days or allow myself one serving a day if I can combine them with *Priority* foods. They taste great but they are calorie dense and don't provide any nutritional benefits.

Avoid Foods:
Processed Foods, Sugar, Trans Fat

Spike Life Food Pyramid
As you noticed, the Spike Life Food Pyramid is upside-down. The foods at the top are the most important and the largest part of the "pyramid." Our food pyramid prioritizes the types of foods that have the biggest weight loss benefits, and limits the foods that can hinder our weight loss goals. The foods we *moderate* and *avoid* should be saved mainly for Spike Days. One day of consuming these types of foods does not inhibit weight loss when the other six days are great. Processed foods like sugar and flour are digested extremely quickly, which results in a high insulin response from the spike in blood sugar. With Spike Life we want to keep our blood sugar stable to keep insulin low and allow glucagon to breakdown and release our fat stores for energy.

CHAPTER 11

CARBOHYDRATES & FIBER

CARBOHYDRATES: THE GOOD, THE BAD, AND THE UGLY

4 Calories per Gram—TEF 6%
(Spike Life Goal: 7-10 Grams per 100 Calories)

At one time, dietary fats were the bad guy, but now carbohydrates have been labeled the new villain of the obesity epidemic. I believe this to be wrong. I heard it said that "sugar is poison," and "carbohydrates make us fat and keep us fat." I personally have debunked that myth and so have other Spikers. I eat carbohydrates and I even have sugar! Somehow, despite that, I've been able to lose over 100 pounds and keep it off. So either I'm not human or carbohydrates are not as evil as some want us to believe. The *no-carb* group does have some valid points, but they miss the most important one and that is: *weight loss is still determined by the Law of Thermodynamics*. I believe it is possible to lose weight on a high-carb diet as long as you keep to a calorie goal that creates a caloric deficit. The problem is it's more difficult to restrict calories on a high-carb plan versus the Spike Life plan.

THE GOOD
Carbohydrates provide good energy

Carbohydrates are our body's favorite fuel source, and they provide us energy for both daily activities and exercise. Carbohydrates are also easily converted to glycogen, stored to be used to fuel our muscles during exercise, and help regulate our blood sugar. Many natural carbohydrate sources are high in fiber and provide a high level satiety per calorie consumed. Fruits and vegetables are very nutrient dense and make us feel fuller on lower calorie amounts.

Foods to eat abundantly:

Vegetables, fruits, "high fiber" foods, and complex carbohydrates like natural oats and whole grains.

> **!** SPIKE LIFE TIP
> Potatoes have gotten a bad rap when it comes to weight loss. Potatoes by themselves are actually very healthy and help you lose weight. They are one of the most filling foods and they are very nutrient-dense.

THE BAD
Carbohydrates have a large impact of blood glucose levels

Since many carbohydrates are easily converted to glucose, they cause our blood sugar to rise rapidly. This is when insulin is released and it begins storing the excess glucose as glycogen. If there are any leftover calories, they are converted to triglycerides and stored as body fat. The other negative is when insulin is released, our body stops burning fat for energy because the fat-burning hormone glucagon cannot coexist with insulin. I call it a *fat-burning switch*. As I am going through the day, my body is consistently burning fat to maintain my metabolism, and then when I begin eating carbohydrates, my blood sugar rises. Then insulin is released and the fat-burning switch goes off. My body begins burning the calories I'm consuming and storing the extra calories I'm not using. For most of us, as long as we are in an overall calorie deficit, then it's not a big deal. We will be burning and storing carbohydrates, body fat, and glycogen all day long, but the overall negative net caloric deficit for a full week will allow us to lose weight consistently.

One of the important goals with Spike Life is keep blood glucose stable. We want to keep insulin levels down so our body will be able to produce more glucagon and burn more body fat. Insulin is more effective the less we use it, and this leads us to the ugly…

Foods to eat in moderation:
Wheat bread, brown rice, whole grain pasta, whole grain cereal.

THE UGLY
Having high amounts of carbohydrates can lead to insulin resistance

Refined carbohydrates like sugar and flour have a greater impact on our blood glucose levels. This is seen on the glycemic index table in this chapter. When we constantly increase our blood sugar levels, insulin gets "overworked," or another word is "tolerant." Kind of like caffeine, the first time you have caffeine, you feel lots of energy. But eventually, after you've had it over and over, you quit feeling the same effects. When insulin is overused, our body quits responding to high and low blood sugar situations like it should. This is what is known as Insulin Resistance or Metabolic Syndrome. Metabolic Syndrome is directly related to obesity and numerous other health problems.

Insulin resistance is when our bodies cannot use insulin effectively. When this happens we can't control the amount of sugar in the body. As a result, blood sugar and fat levels rise. This is the main reason why carbohydrates are demonized. People who are insulin resistant struggle to lose and maintain weight, and it greatly increases the risk for Type 2 Diabetes and Coronary Artery Disease.

Foods to eat sparingly:

Sugar, high fructose corn syrup, white starches, processed foods.

CARBOHYDRATES AND THE GI INDEX

It's probable that if we were to just quit consuming carbohydrates, especially processed carbohydrates, that we would all be healthier and obesity would drop dramatically. The problem is, I don't think it's realistic to live in our society and not consume carbohydrates. Carbs are everywhere and in almost everything, and despite the negative abuse, carbohydrates have positive factors too. Carbs are great for exercise because they are easily stored as glycogen. Most naturally high carbohydrate foods contain fiber which can help us lose weight. Last but not least, carbs just taste so darn good! I'm a "carb person." I couldn't imagine never eating bread, pizza, ice cream, or donuts ever again. I wouldn't want to give them up forever, even for the most ripped physique on the planet.

The real issue isn't carbohydrates themselves. It's the impact they have on blood glucose and then insulin that is the true problem. The good news is that by eating the Spike Life way, we can have our carbohydrates and still keep our blood glucose stable most of the time.

There is a Glycemic Index (GI) chart in this book. This chart gives foods a rating on how they affect our fasting blood glucose levels. The higher the number, the more they increase our blood sugar. Apples are very low on the glycemic index, because the sugar (fructose) is bound with fiber, which slows the absorption. However, apple juice has double the glycemic load as a whole apple because the fiber has been removed.

This chart simply shows how these foods affect our fasting glucose levels; the higher the number, the greater the impact on our blood sugar. However, this chart doesn't tell the whole story.

Glycemic Load

Like the glycemic index, the glycemic load of a food is used to estimate its effect on blood sugar. A food may have a high glycemic index, meaning the carbohydrates it contains quickly convert to sugar, but if that food contains fiber and not many carbohydrates per average serving, there will be less of an impact on blood sugar. A great example of this is watermelon. It has a high glycemic index of 103 but a low glycemic load of 4. So even though the GI says it will increase your blood sugar, it actually will not.

GLYCEMIC INDEX (GI) CHART

	FOOD	GLYCEMIC INDEX
Sugars	Maltose	105
	Glucose	100
	Sucrose (table sugar)	65
	Honey	58
	Lactose (milk)	46
	Agave Nectar	30
	Fructose (fruit)	23
Starches	Bagel	72
	White Bread	70
	Whole Wheat Bread	69
	Sourdough Bread	52
	Sponge Cake	46
Fruits	Watermelon	103
	Pineapple	66
	Cantaloupe	65
	Banana	55
	Grapes	46
	Orange	44
	Apple	38
	Cherries	22

GI < 55 = Low, GI 55-70 = Intermediate, GI > 70 = High

Calculating Glycemic Load

To calculate the glycemic load of a food, multiply GI by the number of digestible (non-fiber) carbohydrates in a single serving, then divide by 100.

GL < 10 = Low
GL 10—19 = Medium
GL > 20 = High

Making Higher GI Foods Have Less of an Impact on Blood Sugar

In looking at meals as a whole, combining high glycemic index foods with protein and fiber slows the absorption of sugar and lessens the overall impact on blood glucose levels.

GI EXAMPLE:		
Instant oatmeal	High GI	Increased blood glucose
Instant oatmeal with strawberries & tsp. of fiber powder	Low GI	Stable blood glucose

When we create our Spike Life meal plans, we want to have a balanced amount of protein, fats, and carbohydrates. Fiber should be included in each meal, and we don't want to have high GI foods on an empty stomach. One of the worst things we can do for breakfast is wake up and consume a highly processed, carbohydrate-rich meal, like cereal. This starts the day off with a blood glucose surge that will result in a subsequent blood glucose crash. This leaves us hungry and lethargic. Instead, our breakfast needs to be high in protein and fiber. This will give us hours of stable energy and keep our hunger away.

BETTER CHOICES FOR HIGH GI CARBOHYDRATES

HIGH GI	SPIKE LIFE "BETTER CHOICES"
White Bread	"Light" Italian Bread
Tortillas	"Low-Carb" White Flour Tortillas
Pizza Crust	"Low-Carb" Flat Breads
Sugar	Agave or Honey
Chocolate	Chocolate Protein Powder
Couscous	Quinoa
Pasta	Shirataki Noodles
Candy Bar	Protein Bar
Ice Cream	Coconut Milk Ice Cream
White Flour	Combination of Almond Flour and Coconut Flour
Yogurt	Greek Yogurt
Smoothies	Kefir

The quicker foods digest the more they affect blood sugar

The general rule of thumb is: the more processed a food is, the quicker it will be digested and increase your blood glucose levels. Living the Spike Life, we want to avoid highly processed foods and choose foods that are more natural and digested slower. The other option is to combine high GI foods with protein and fiber to slow the digestion.

Dealing with Carb Cravings

I am a "carb person," I love breads and sweets. While I am able to tame my cravings with Spike Day, I still find myself wanting them during the other six days. It's not that carbohydrates are bad, it's just they are high in calories, can increase insulin, and often lack nutrients we actually need. Choosing "high-fiber" or "low-carb" options can curb cravings while providing us a nutritional benefit. So I have found ways to replace high carbohydrate foods with healthier choices.

THE SNACK FOOD DIET

To test of the rule of *calories in versus calories out equals weight loss*, Mark Haub, a professor of human nutrition at Kansas State University, chose to embark on his weight loss journey by eating Twinkies! He ate one Twinkie every three hours, instead of meals. To add variety, he also ate Hostess and Little Debbie snack cakes, Doritos chips, sugary cereals, and Oreos. He limited his daily calories to 1,800 a day and he lost 27 lbs in two months. He proved that for short-term weight loss, calories in versus calories out are what matters most and not the nutritional value of the food.

I do not recommend this for long-term weight loss

While Haub did lose 27 lbs in two months, the snack food diet is something I would definitely not recommend. Sure, calories are more important than the nutritional value, but that's because it's a law of nature. This doesn't mean nutritional value isn't important, because it is. I don't see how living this way would work long-term, which is the goal of Spike Life. I would imagine days full of physical hunger and mental breakdowns. I believe choosing to eat this way leaves a very slim chance of keeping the weight off. He did, however, prove a point. Regardless of what the low-carb proponents say, you can lose weight eating a high-carb diet. Overall, it's calories in versus out that determines weight loss and or weight gain.

FIBER

0-4 Calories per Gram—High Fiber Carbohydrates TEF 20% (Spike Life Goal: 2-3 Grams per 100 Calories)

Fiber is listed as a carbohydrate on food labels, but it's either not digestible or slowly digested. Often you will see a mention on a food label of "net-carbs"; this is the carbohydrate total subtracted by the fiber content. Fiber is found naturally in fruits, vegetables, and whole grains. Having fiber with each meal is an important part of living the Spike Life.

In 2003, the World Health Organization made the statement that there is "convincing evidence" showing that dietary fiber aids in protecting us against weight gain and obesity. Fiber has the ability to increase satiety and therefore decrease our cravings and hunger. Fiber can help control our blood sugar by slowing the absorption of high glycemic-load foods, and lessen the impact of those foods and our blood glucose levels. Fiber helps to stabilize our blood sugar and lessen the impact of insulin. This is important for both diabetics and those of us trying to control our weight.

A high-fiber diet has many benefits, including:

- High-fiber foods help us control our weight because they tend to make us feel full longer, so we are less likely to feel the need to constantly snack.
- High-fiber foods are less "energy dense," which means they have fewer calories for the same volume of food.
- Helps control blood sugar levels. Soluble fiber can slow the absorption of sugar. A diet that includes insoluble fiber has been associated with a reduced risk of developing type 2 diabetes.
- Helps maintain bowel integrity and health.
- For some, fiber may provide relief from irritable bowel syndrome.
- A high-fiber diet may lower your risk of developing hemorrhoids.
- Some fiber is fermented in the colon; this may help prevent disease in the colon.
- Lowers blood cholesterol levels. Soluble fiber found in beans, oats, flaxseed, and oat bran may help lower total blood cholesterol levels by lowering (LDL) low-density lipoprotein, or "bad," cholesterol levels.
- Increased fiber in the diet can reduce blood pressure and inflammation, which is also protective to heart health.

THE THREE MAIN TYPES OF DIETARY FIBER
Insoluble fiber, soluble fiber and resistant starch

INSOLUBLE FIBER
Insoluble fibers keep their shape in water. They promote the movement of foods through your digestive system and provide bulking in foods without adding extra calories.

Foods high in Insoluble Fiber include:
- Whole Grains
- Whole Wheat Flour
- Wheat Bran
- Nuts
- Vegetables

SOLUBLE FIBER
Some soluble fibers lose their shape when mixed in water. They reduce cholesterol absorption and contribute to colon health by increasing intestinal fermentation. This leads to better digestive health.

Foods high in Soluble Fiber include:

- ▶ Inulin
- ▶ Oat Bran
- ▶ Parsnips
- ▶ Peas
- ▶ Potatoes
- ▶ Lentils
- ▶ Beans

RESISTANT STARCH

Some resistant starches reduce the glycemic load of foods and also contribute to colon and metabolic system health. Resistant starches also increase lipid metabolism and improve insulin sensitivity.

Foods high in Resistant Starch include:

- ▶ Unripe Bananas
- ▶ Corn
- ▶ Potatoes
- ▶ Yams
- ▶ Pasta
- ▶ Barley
- ▶ Whole Grain Bread
- ▶ Navy Beans
- ▶ Oatmeal
- ▶ Lentils
- ▶ Brown Rice

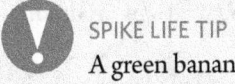 SPIKE LIFE TIP
A green banana contains 12.5 grams of resistant starch.

FIBER CAN HELP YOU LOSE WEIGHT

The research has shown that fiber and resistant starch foods can shrink fat cells, increase muscle mass, curb cravings, and keep people feeling full for longer. It is obvious that all types of fiber can aid in weight loss and overall health. This is why fiber is extremely important to living the Spike Life. Fiber is right along with protein as the most important nutrients to losing and maintaining weight loss. The American Dietetic Association recommends adults 20-35 grams of fiber daily. The average American only gets 14-15 grams daily. For living the Spike Life, I recommend that we get 30-50 grams of fiber daily, and I practice what I preach. My goal is to have at least 10 grams of fiber with every meal, and then I may supplement my diet with natural fiber powder or snack on high fiber foods.

My favorite high fiber foods:
- ▶ Fruits
- ▶ Vegetables
- ▶ High Fiber Breads (many "light" breads have less calories but extra fiber)
- ▶ Oat Bran and 100% Whole Grain Bread
- ▶ High Fiber Tortillas
- ▶ High Fiber Flatbreads
- ▶ Fiber Bars
- ▶ Fiber Yogurt
- ▶ Tasteless Natural Fiber Powder (supplement)

Ways to supplement with pure and tasteless fiber powder
- ▶ Add fiber to ice water
- ▶ Protein Shakes
- ▶ Mix it in sauces
- ▶ On top of meals
- ▶ Add it to peanut butter
- ▶ Mix in yogurt

Each heaping teaspoon of fiber powder contains about 5 grams of soluble fiber

Ways to Increase Fiber Daily
While the average American is well below the Spike Life recommended daily amount of fiber, it is actually extremely easy to get there by choosing the right foods and using supplements to make up the difference.

Most "low-carb" or "high-fiber" tortillas have 7-12 grams of fiber, compared to one or zero for regular tortillas. "Light" breads contain about 4-6 grams per serving, compared to one or zero for regular white or wheat bread. Vegetables and fruits also contain a high amount of fiber per calorie. If you have been one of the many consuming too little fiber, it is a good idea to slowly increase your fiber intake, for example; if you have been having only 15 grams daily in the past. I would start with 20 grams the first week, 25 grams week two, 30 grams weeks three, and so on until you are averaging 35-50 grams of fiber daily. If you significantly increase your fiber intake too quick, it can lead to stomach pains and gas.

A TYPICAL SPIKE LIFE DAY FOR FIBER INTAKE:

MEAL	FOODS	FIBER
Breakfast	Eggs and fruit. Water w/Fiber Powder	10 grams
Snack	Fiber Bar	5 grams
Lunch	Grilled Chicken & Veggies	8 grams
Snack	Greek Yogurt w/Fiber Powder	7 grams
Dinner	Chicken Enchiladas w/Corn and "High-Fiber" Tortillas	24 grams
Snack	Cheese Stick	0

Total Fiber for the Day: 54 grams

CARBOHYDRATES AND FIBER SUMMARY:

Carbohydrates are not as evil as some think; as you have read, they too have their role in living the Spike Life. I recommend we get 33% of our daily calories from carbohydrates and 30-50 grams of fiber. We should avoid eating highly processed foods and focus on the natural choices of carbohydrates.

CHAPTER 12

FAT

DIETARY FAT

9 Calories per Gram—TEF 3%
(Spike Life Goal: 3-4 Grams per 100 Calories)

Dietary fat is a victim of guilt by name association. When I was young I assumed, like many people do, that eating fat makes you fat. What I know now is that overall calories are what really matters and that dietary fat can actually help us lose weight. In fact, without essential fats, losing weight and keeping it off would be extremely difficult.

For many years health professionals believed that saturated fats were the cause of heart disease. In recent years studies have been conducted in regions where highly saturated fats such as coconut oil and palm oil are consumed. In most of those regions, meat and dairy are also regularly consumed. The researchers found that in those populations, heart disease is very rare. They discovered that the main cause of heart disease is actually excessive consumption of trans fats and refined carbohydrates such as processed flour and sugars. Natural fats are extremely important for hormone production and vitamin absorption. The only fat that can be truly called unhealthy is trans fat.

Dietary fat does not make you fat!

Dietary fat has been wrongly demonized by the medical community for making us overweight, raising cholesterol, and causing heart disease. This is false; in fact, there hasn't been one study showing a correlation between saturated fat and heart disease. It is true the elevated triglycerides (fats) in the blood have been positively linked to heart disease, but these triglycerides do not come directly from dietary fats. Triglycerides are made in the liver from any excess sugars (glucose) that have not been used for energy. The source of these *excess* sugars is any food containing carbohydrates, particularly refined sugar and white flour like pasta, breads, and rice. Or what Arnold Schwarzenegger called the "White Death" back in the 1970s when his life depended upon his ability to terminate body fat.

The facts are we need dietary fat. There are essential fatty acids that we cannot survive without. One of the keys to living the Spike Life is giving our body what it needs. If we satisfy the needs of our body, we are less likely to have uncontrollable food cravings and our body is able to work the way it is supposed to work.

What are some signs you are not eating enough dietary fat?

- Low testosterone in males
- Chronic degenerative diseases such as: arthritis, coronary artery disease, high blood pressure, osteoporosis, stroke
- Type 2 diabetes
- Constipation
- Dry, itchy, scaly skin, including cracked fingers and heels
- Fat around the middle and an overall flabby body
- Infertility
- Malnutrition
- Brittle nails and dry, thinning hair
- Insomnia and extreme fatigue
- Mood swings, depression, and other emotional disorders
- Sugar and stimulant cravings

 SPIKE LIFE TIP

Dietary fats are needed to produce key sex hormones that promote healthy weight and anti-aging.

Spike Life Fats to Prioritize

- Omega-3s
- Lauric Acid
- Oleic Acid

POLYSATURATED FATTY ACIDS

These fats improve blood cholesterol levels and may also help decrease the risk of type 2 diabetes. Our essential fats are polyunsaturated fats.

Oils high in polyunsaturated fatty acids are:

- Corn
- Safflower
- Soybean
- Sesame
- Sunflower Seed Oil
- Seafood

ESSENTIAL FATTY ACIDS (EFAS)
Omega-3s and Omega-6s

OMEGA-3 FATTY ACIDS—SPIKE PRIORITY FAT

Omega-3s are an essential polyunsaturated fat. Omega-3 fatty acids can help to reduce inflammation, raise good HDL cholesterol, and reduce triglycerides.

Foods that is high in omega-3s are:
- Grass-Fed Beef
- Farm Fresh Eggs
- Anchovies
- Salmon
- Sardines
- Tuna
- Mackerel
- Walnuts
- Canola Oil
- Flaxseed Oil

OMEGA-6 FATTY ACIDS

Omega-6s are also a polyunsaturated fat, but many Americans get them in abundance with processed oils and meat. They are essential and our health would suffer without them, but it's important to our health to stay within the 4:1 ratio of omega-6s to omega-3s. While omega-3 fatty acids can help to reduce inflammation, most omega-6 fatty acids tend to promote inflammation.

Foods that are high in Omega-6 fatty acids are:
- Fish
- Dairy fat
- Walnuts
- Flaxseed oil
- Hemp seed oil
- Pumpkin seed oil
- Sesame seed oil
- Evening primrose oil

OTHER NON-ESSENTIAL FATS WITH HEALTH BENEFITS
Monounsaturated Fats and Saturated Fats

MONOUNSATURATED FATTY ACIDS

Studies show that eating foods rich in monounsaturated fats helps to improve blood cholesterol levels. They may also be beneficial to insulin levels and blood sugar control.

Oils that are high in monounsaturated fatty acids are:

▶ Olives
▶ Canola
▶ Nut Oils

OLEIC ACID—SPIKE PRIORITY FAT

Also known as omega-9 fatty acid, oleic acid is a monounsaturated fatty acid that is essential to our health. However, it is considered a nonessential fat because our body can make it in limited amounts when other essential fatty acids are available. Oleic acid lowers the risk of a heart attack by reducing LDL cholesterol.

Foods that are high in oleic acid are:

▶ Avocados
▶ Macadamia Nuts
▶ Apricot Seeds
▶ Almonds
▶ Olive Oil
▶ Grape Seed Oil
▶ Nuts
▶ Sunflower Oil

SATURATED FATTY ACIDS

Many people believe that saturated fat causes heart disease. The truth is there is no evidence that saturated fat or cholesterol-rich foods cause heart disease. My belief is that overeating in general causes obesity and heart disease. When glycogen storage is at capacity, excess calories are converted to triglycerides and are sent through our blood to be stored as body fat. The combination of inflammation in the arteries, LDL cholesterol, and triglycerides are the biggest issues for heart disease. Following the Spike Life, I don't want you to be afraid of natural saturated fats. I ate them when I lost 100 lbs and I still do today. Staying within your calorie range is what you need to focus on.

Foods high in saturated fatty acids are:
- Red Meats
- Poultry
- Butter
- Whole Milk
- Tropical Oils

LAURIC ACID—SPIKE PRIORITY FAT

Lauric acid is a saturated fat that promotes health by fighting bacteria and viruses. It can also fight heart disease by lowering LDL (bad) cholesterol.

Foods that are high in Lauric acid are:
- Coconuts
- Coconut Oil
- Palm Kernel Oil

> **SPIKE LIFE TIP**
> Coconut oil is mostly saturated fat, but it's a unique type of fat called MCTs or medium-chain-triglycerides. MCTs are sent directly to the liver and converted to energy and cannot be stored as body fat. They can actually stimulate our metabolism and help us lose weight. They are also being used to treat Alzheimer's and dementia because they provide immediate backup energy for our brain. Coconut oil is the best kind of fat for health and losing weight. Since coconut oil is great for high-heat use, I use it to cook, fry, and bake my meals.

THE ONE FAT TO AVOID—TRANS FATTY ACIDS

Trans fatty acids are formed during the process of hydrogenation. The hydrogenated fats are actually unsaturated fats which have been processed to make them solid and stable at room temperature. Hydrogenated fats were created for the purpose of extending shelf life on packaged foods so they could last longer and be cheaper to the consumer. They are wrongly called "healthier" than natural sources because they contain less saturated fat and have the word "vegetable" attached to them. Check food labels and avoid any food that has hydrogenated fats or oils of any kind.

Sources containing trans fatty acids include:

▶ Margarine
▶ Shortening
▶ Processed and packaged foods such as crackers and cookies.

Trans Fatty Acids and Cholesterol

Trans fats raise bad blood cholesterol levels (LDL), and lower good HDL levels. Trans fats are **not** essential and they do **not** promote health. Foods containing trans fats need to be limited to Spike Days and kept at an absolute minimum. Since most processed foods also contain high levels of processed carbohydrates, these foods contain the *double whammy* of raising triglycerides levels in our blood, and lowering the HDL cholesterol that would pick them up and carry them away. Trans fats can lead to clogged arteries and heart disease.

COCONUT OIL—SPIKE PREFERRED FAT

Coconut oil is my fat of choice. I consume 2-3 Tbsp of coconut oil daily, and the health benefits go beyond weight loss.

Coconut oil contains a very high amount of lauric acid and the highest natural amount of MCT, medium chain triglycerides. What makes (MCT) medium chain triglycerides unique is that MCTs bypass stomach metabolism and go directly to your liver where they are converted into ketones. The liver then immediately releases the ketones into the bloodstream where they are transported to the brain to be used as fuel. It is impossible for MCTs to be converted to body fat, making coconut oil a dietary fat that cannot make you fat.

Research has shown that the ketone bodies produced by MCTs provide a stable source of energy for the brain during periods of low blood sugar, without the neurological risks associated with high blood sugar. This is very important because if you are limiting your calories in an attempt to lose weight, there could be periods of time when your blood sugar is low and stored glycogen in you liver could also be low. This can cause you to feel hypoglycemic.

The Fat that Helps You Lose Weight

Back in the 1940s farmers started using coconut oil in an attempt to fatten up their livestock; amazingly, the opposite happened. Their livestock not only lost weight, but their energy levels increased, too. This was potentially brought on by coconut oil's effect on our thyroid and how it regulates metabolism.

The truth about coconut oil is obvious to anyone who has studied its health benefits but yet it has remained a *diet secret* to most in the mainstream. But why?

That's a great question. Coconut oil used to be used in our movie theatre popcorn, but then it happened! Saturated Fat become the root all of things dietary evil. Well, since coconut oil is over 90% saturated fat, it was burned at the stake just like all the other "healthy natural fats" during the "Heart Disease Witch Hunt" of the 1970s. Coconut oil was replaced by partially hydrogenated vegetable oils—since it's vegetable fat, it must be healthier, right?

Wrong!

Partially hydrogenated oils contain trans fats, and according to the Mayo Clinic and everyone else, trans fat is considered to be the worst type of fat. Unlike other fats, trans fat—also called trans fatty acids—both raises your "bad" (LDL) cholesterol and lowers your "good" (HDL) cholesterol.

The easiest way to remember this: HDL is good cholesterol, we want it high (H), and LDL is the bad cholesterol, we want it low (L).

I also felt it was strange that, for the longest time, the only place I could buy coconut oil was health food stores! If it is so bad for me because of the saturated fat, why is it sold in health food stores? Isn't that a direct contradiction? Coconut oil was wrongly demonized by the mainstream because of its high saturated fat content, but it is quickly making a comeback. It is, in my opinion, the healthiest fat and the most beneficial for weight loss.

Medium chain triglycerides found in coconut oil are good for you

▶ They improve your heart health by increasing HDL Cholesterol
▶ Boost your thyroid production
▶ Increase your metabolism and energy output
▶ Promote a lean body and weight loss if needed
▶ Support your immune system
▶ Provide your brain with energy. It's the "Ultimate Brain Food"
▶ Are anti-microbial
▶ Help with weight loss, improves skin ailments, and ulcers
▶ Help to treat ulcers by killing off H Pylori bacteria

Go to spikelifebook.com to get a full list of the health benefits of coconut oil

How to Use Coconut Oil in Your Diet

I use both virgin and expelled pressed coconut oil; the difference is the expelled pressed removes the coconut smell and taste so it will not affect the flavor of foods that I add it to. I use coconut oil both for frying foods, in baking, and just as a topper, much like you would use butter on top of toast.

Now you might be thinking that since most of the calories in coconut oil cannot be stored as fat, then it's a "free food" and you can eat as much as you want. Well, unfortunately, that is not true. Really, there is no such thing as a free food or a *negative calorie* food. Even though MCTs can't be stored as fat, studies show that *when we burn one type of fuel we burn less of another.* So while we are burning fats for energy, we are burning fewer carbohydrates, and when we are burning carbohydrate calories, we are burning fewer fat calories. This goes back to the Law of Thermodynamics; this is exactly why total calories consumption is what truly matters. So we definitely still need to count the calories we consume from coconut oil, as they are included in our daily energy balance.

Cooking with Coconut Oil

- ▶ Use as a spread instead of butter
- ▶ Baking; saturated fats are great for high heat use
- ▶ Add to protein shakes
- ▶ Use as an oil for frying foods
- ▶ Make "healthier desserts"
- ▶ Microwave 1 Tbsp of coconut oil with a handful of chocolate chips for thirty seconds for a healthier chocolate topping. It hardens like a chocolate shell on top of ice cream and cold fruits

> **! SPIKE LIFE TIP**
> Coconut oil is great for skin and hair! Lauric acids fight off fungal infections, and can treat psoriasis and emphysema.

WHERE'S THE BEEF...FROM?
Grass-Fed Beef vs. Grain-Fed Beef

The way animals are raised and fed effects the quality of the meat we consume. Grass-fed beef is lower in overall fat and calories than grain-fed cattle. Grass-fed beef also contains higher levels of essential omega-3 fatty acids and CLA (conjugated linoleic acid).

Omega-3

Scientific studies have shown that when our omega-6 to omega-3 exceeds 4:1, people have more health problems. This is important because grain-fed beef has an omega-6 to omega-3 ratio of 20:1, while grass-fed is 3:1.

CLA

Grass-fed beef is great natural source of CLA (conjugated linoleic acid), a fat that reduces the risk of cancer, obesity, diabetes, and a number of immune disorders.

Benefits of Choosing Grass-Fed Beef:
- ▶ Grass-fed beef has the recommended ratio of omega-6 to omega-3 fats (3:1)
- ▶ Loaded with vitamins and minerals
- ▶ Natural source of CLA
- ▶ Fewer calories and less overall fat
- ▶ Grass is the natural food for cattle

Grass-fed beef is a Spike Life Priority Food. You can find fresh and frozen extra lean cuts of hamburger, steak, and other beef products in most grocery stores. You can also search out local farms that sell grass-fed beef and other pasture raised meats.

DIETARY FATS WHILE LIVING THE SPIKE LIFE

Fats to prioritize
- ▶ Lauric acid
- ▶ Omega-3s
- ▶ Oleic acid

Fats to enjoy
- ▶ Omega-6s
- ▶ Monounsaturated fat
- ▶ Polyunsaturated fat

Fat to keep in moderation
- ▶ Saturated Fats (*Exception is coconut oil*)

Fats to avoid
- ▶ Trans fats
- ▶ Hydrogenated oils
- ▶ Partially hydrogenated oils

DIETARY FAT SUMMARY:

We need good natural fats in our diet. Almost every type of dietary fat has health benefits, other than of trans fats. Healthy dietary fats will help you lose weight and live a healthier life. For Spike Life, I recommend we get 33% of our daily calories from fat, but we need to focus on natural fats and not the processed ones.

CHAPTER 13

THE POWER OF PROTEIN

PROTEIN ESSENTIALS

4 Calories per Gram—TEF 30-35%
(SPIKE LIFE GOAL: 7-10 GRAMS PER 100 CALORIES)

Proteins are organic compounds made of amino acids arranged in a linear chain, and as you probably learned in science class, amino acids are the building blocks for life. Amino acids are what our body uses to build muscle, hair, nails, skin, our immune system, metabolism, and much more. When we exercise our body needs more protein than the average person, and a shortage of amino acids is devastating to what would be a successful diet and workout program.

Protein is the most important nutrient for weight loss

Like I said before, not every calorie was created equal. If there was a competition for the best calorie for weight loss, protein would win in a landslide. Besides being an essential nutrient, protein has three important weight loss benefits.

The Weight Loss Benefits of Protein:

▸ Protein has a high level of satiety
▸ Protein boosts our metabolism because it has by far the highest thermic effect (TEF)
▸ Protein helps us build and maintain muscle

Protein makes us feel full!

Hunger is always an issue for those of us trying to lose weight. Protein has a high satiety level, this one reason is why we need to consume protein with every meal.

Protein Boosts Our Metabolism!

Another great attribute of protein is its thermogenic effect. While losing weight is as simple as calories in versus calories out, not all calories are created equal. Eating in general increases metabolism in the short term but, because protein has to be broken down into amino acids, almost 30% of the calories eaten have to be used in the digestion of the protein. For example, if you have something with 40 grams of protein, which is 160 calories, 50 of those calories will be burned up in the process of digesting the food. This is on top of your calories burned through BMR and activities.

Protein Helps Us Build and Maintain Muscle!

Building strength and muscle is extremely important to long-term weight loss and our health. We burn more calories daily when we increase our muscle or lean body mass. Our body uses protein to build muscle and maintain their strength. If we don't get enough protein, we run the risk of losing muscle mass, which lowers our metabolism.

How Much Protein do you Need?

Personally, I got my best results when I ate one gram of protein multiplied by my body weight. For example, I weigh 215 lbs so I eat about 215 grams of protein a day, which I find to be sufficient for my recovery. The general rule is the more intense the weight training, the more protein you need.

Simply multiply your weight in pounds by one of the following:

▸ Sedentary adult: 0.4 gram per pound
▸ Active adult: 0.4-0.6 gram per pound
▸ Athletes and Building Strength: 0.6-0.9 gram per pound
▸ Living the Spike Life: 0.6-1 gram per pound

(These are all estimates for healthy adults and may not be appropriate for people with chronic kidney disease, liver disease, or diabetes. Please see your physician for nutritional advice if you have these conditions. I believe you need to find the correct amount for you. For myself, I produced my best results after I increased my protein intake.)

AMINO ACIDS

Proteins look like long strings with differently shaped spheres. Each sphere is a small amino acid. These amino acids can be bonded together, called peptides, to make thousands of different proteins. All proteins are made up of some combination of amino acids. Individual proteins, for example: whey and soy proteins contain different numbers and proportions of amino acids. This is why it's good to get your proteins from a wide variety of sources.

Amino Acids

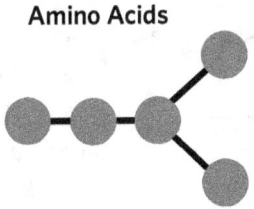

Scientists have found many different amino acids in protein, but twenty of them are very important to human health. Of those twenty amino acids, your body can actually create ten of them. Your body can't make the other ten amino acids, but you can get them by eating protein-rich foods. They are called essential amino acids because they are *essential* to our health, and you can only get them from the foods you eat. Failure to obtain enough of just one of the ten essential amino acids results in breakdown of proteins from our muscles to obtain the one amino acid that is needed. Unlike fat and glycogen (carbohydrates), the human body does not store excess amino acids for later use. The only way to for our body to get amino acids is from the foods we eat and cannibalizing muscle tissue using the catabolic hormones, cortisol and glucagon. Since losing muscle tissue will result in a lower metabolism and loss of strength, it is extremely important to the Spike Life that we get amino acids in our meals everyday.

The ten essential amino acids:
- Arginine, classified as "semi-essential"
- Histidine
- Isoleucine
- Leucine
- Lysine
- Methionine
- Phenylalanine
- Threonine
- Tryptophan
- Valine

We can get our essential amino acids from eating a well-balanced diet of lean meats, dairy, grains, and vegetables. You can also supplement with protein powders to make sure you get all of the amino acids you need.

PROTEIN SOURCES & BIOLOGICAL VALUE

PROTEIN SOURCES & BIOLOGICAL VALUE	
PROTEIN	**BIOLOGICAL VALUE (BV)**
Whey Protein Isolate	100-159
Whole Egg	100
Milk	91
Fish	82
Beef	80
Chicken	79
Soy	74
Casein	71

Values are approximate. Whey Isolate is the highest quality protein.

Every protein source has a biological value (BV). The BV of a protein source indicates how fully the body absorbs and utilizes the protein. The higher the value, the more completely the protein consumed will be absorbed and used by the body. The chart below gives the BV* of common protein sources.

113

TYPES OF PROTEINS:

Whey Protein

Whey protein is quickly digested and absorbed into the body with the highest biological value of 105-150 on the scale. It is the most utilized form of protein, has very little lactose, and is typically very easy on your digestive system.

WHEN TO USE: It is best taken in the morning, after a night of fasting, to get a quick supply of amino acids to your muscles. It is also a benefit to use whey protein after lifting weights for maximum results.

Egg Protein

Egg Protein is great for muscle building and endurance training with its high biological value (100). Egg protein was the benchmark for all proteins before whey protein was introduced. It can be taken at any time during the day. When to use: I highly recommend it at night, before bed, mixed with other proteins, as it will provide protein through the night.

Milk (Casein) Protein

Casein protein is a naturally time-released protein. It has a high BV and is often mixed in meal replacement protein powders.

WHEN TO USE: Like egg protein, this is my favorite before bed protein supplement.

Buckwheat Protein

Buckwheat Protein is my favorite vegetarian alternative to milk and egg proteins. It's naturally rich in key amino acids including arginine, glutamine, and leucine, and free of lactose and cholesterol.

WHEN TO USE: Buckwheat protein is easily is the best alternative for vegetarians as a daily protein supplement.

Soy Protein

Soy protein is easily absorbed by your body; it helps lower bad cholesterol, it's lactose free, and is a good alternative for vegetarians.

WHEN TO USE: Soy protein is quickly absorbed, making it good post-workout. I recommend using soy sparingly.

Protein to avoid:

Gelatin is a protein usually listed as *Hydrolyzed Collagen* in many supplements, including protein bars and drinks. It is the lowest quality protein with a BV of near zero. Look out for that ingredient in protein supplements before buying them.

Calories still count!

Remember to stay within your daily calorie goal. If you eat more protein, you will need to consume less carbohydrates and fats. It is very important to consume protein post-workout. The best protein after you workout is in the form of a whey isolate. You can usually buy these in ready-to-drink bottles at your gym. You can also purchase whey protein powders from most grocery stores and mix them with water or milk. Whey protein is the best because it is the most easily absorbed and the quickest to get to your broken-down muscle tissue. It's important to get protein from multiple sources because they all contain different amounts of essential amino acids. Sources include lean red meat, pork, poultry, fish, eggs, vegetables, and milk products. These proteins are not as easily absorbed as pure whey, but they can provide a wealth of amino acids for your body for several hours. Having a mix of slower digesting proteins are great to consume before going to bed to provide amino acids for your body while you are sleeping.

FOODS TO EAT: Grass-fed beef, protein supplements, extra lean red meats like 93/7 ground beef, fish, poultry, nuts, milk, and eggs.

Spike Life uses for protein powders

▶ Post-workout: whey protein shake for fast absorption and availability.
▶ Use a blended protein powder as a meal replacement for a longer, more sustained release of amino acids.
▶ Slow digesting protein like casein before bed.
▶ Mix protein with peanut butter for a delicious snack.
▶ Breading in place of flour. Add spices to unflavored protein powder, and then dip chicken in liquid egg whites and roll in spiced protein powder.
▶ Add protein powder to pancake mix, flour, muffins, and other baked goods.
▶ Homemade ice cream!
▶ No-Bake bars and fudge.

PROTEIN SUMMARY:

Protein is the most beneficial type of calorie we can consume for fat-burning. It has the highest thermic effect on metabolism, it helps to stabilize blood sugar, and it provides a high level of satiety. Protein is a priority while living the Spike Life. I recommend we get 34% of our daily calories from proteins.

MY FAVORITE PROTEIN POWDER RECIPES:

"Protein Power" Recipes
- ▶ Chewy No-Bake Oatmeal Protein Bars
- ▶ Protein Power Pancakes
- ▶ Protein Power Fudge
- ▶ Protein Power Ice Cream
- ▶ Protein Power Chocolate Peanut Butter Wraps
- ▶ Protein Power Cake Batter Bowls

CHEWY NO-BAKE OATMEAL PROTEIN BARS
(Makes 12 bars)

Ingredients:

3 Cups rolled oats

2 Scoops natural vanilla protein powder

¼ Cup pure fiber powder (tasteless)

½ Cup natural peanut butter

¼ Cup agave light syrup

¼ Cup milk

½ Cup expelled pressed coconut oil

½ Cup milk chocolate chips

Instructions:

- ▶ Combine the dry ingredients (oats, 1 scoop of protein, fiber, 1/4 cup of chocolate chips) in small bowl
- ▶ Put peanut butter and agave in a microwave safe bowl, and microwave for 30 seconds
- ▶ Microwave 1/4 cup of coconut oil in a small glass bowl for 30 seconds, or until liquefied
- ▶ Mix peanut butter, agave, and 1 scoop of protein powder until smooth
- ▶ In a large bowl, combine dry ingredients with wet ingredients in small increments
- ▶ Add warmed coconut oil to large bowl and mix well
- ▶ Move to a greased pie pan or small bread pan
- ▶ Press and pack down mixture with a large spoon
- ▶ Refrigerate bars for 30-60 minutes

Instructions for chocolate topping:

- ▶ In a small glass bowl, put 1/4 cup of coconut oil
- ▶ Add 1/4 cup of milk chocolate chips
- ▶ Microwave for 35 seconds
- ▶ Stir together and set aside
- ▶ When bars have cooled, drizzle chocolate sauce over top
- ▶ Cool bars for 15-20 more minutes
- ▶ Cut into equal sizes, makes about 12 bars

Nutrition Information:

- ▶ Per Bar (about 4x2 inches)
- ▶ 275 Calories

- ▶ 10g Fat (about 3 grams of fat from MCT oil)
- ▶ 28g Carbs
- ▶ 8g Fiber
- ▶ 18g Protein

PROTEIN POWER PANCAKES

The taste reminds me of a "French Toast Pancake" and my very picky kids love them.

Ingredients

  1 Scoop natural vanilla protein powder
  ½ Cup egg liquid substitute
  ½ tsp baking powder
  ½ Tbsp expelled pressed coconut oil

Directions:

  ▶ Warm the coconut oil in microwave safe bowl for 20 seconds or until liquefied
  ▶ Whisk all of the ingredients together. Spray frying pan with non-stick spray
  ▶ Cook in pan until golden brown
  ▶ Top pancakes with 2 Tbsp sugar-free syrup

Nutrition Information:

  ▶ 200 Calories
  ▶ 8g Fat
  ▶ 3g Carbs
  ▶ 27g Protein

PROTEIN POWER PEANUT BUTTER FUDGE

Very quick and easy, no bake, low carb peanut butter fudge bars.
(Makes 9 large bars)

Picture

Ingredients:

  7 Scoops chocolate protein powder
  ½ CupPB2 Powder Peanut Butter*
  ½ Cup expeller pressed coconut oil
  4 Tbsp low-fat cream cheese
  ½ Cup low-fat pasteurized liquid eggs

Directions:

- In a large mixing bowl, combine dry ingredients and mix together with a fork
- Warm coconut oil to a liquid in microwave for 20 seconds
- Warm cream cheese in microwave for 20 seconds
- Add the oil, eggs, and cream cheese to dry mixture and combine with a wooden spoon or spatula
- This is a bit of a forearm workout; mix for about 2-3 minutes
- Place wax paper in a small square pan and spray with non-stick spray
- Pour mix into pan and form with a spoon or spatula
- Refrigerate fudge for 30 minutes
- Cut into 9 equal squares and enjoy

Nutrition Information per Bar:

- 233 Calories
- 16g Fat (Mostly from MCTs in the coconut oil)
- 2g Carbs
- 20g Protein

SPIKE LIFE TIP
PB2 is a natural low-fat powder peanut butter found at bellplantation.com

PROTEIN POWER ICE CREAM

All you need is one large and one small zipping storage bag
(Makes 1 cup of ice cream)

Picture
Ingredients

   1 Scoop protein powder
   ¼ Cup half and half
   ¼ Cup low-fat pasteurized liquid eggs
   ½ Cup milk
   ¼ Cup salt

Directions

   ▶ Fill large bag half full of ice and add salt
   ▶ Put remaining ingredients in the small bag and lock·   Place small bag
     in the large bag with the ice and salt
   ▶ Shake the bags for 5-10 minutes
   ▶ It's a bit of a pre-snack workout!

Nutrition Information:
(Depends on protein powder)

   ▶ 180 Calories
   ▶ 6g Fat
   ▶ 5g Carbs
   ▶ 28g Protein

PROTEIN POWER CAKE BATTER BOWL

Picture

Ingredients:

1 Scoop protein powder

½ Tbsp coconut oil

½ Cup low-fat pasteurized liquid eggs

Directions:

▶ Warm coconut oil to a liquid for 30 seconds in microwave.   In a bowl, add protein and liquid eggs

▶ Mix with spoon for about 10 seconds until smooth

▶ Add oil and mix again

▶ You can eat it right then, or I like to chill it for about 20 minutes.

Nutrition Info:

(*Depends on protein powder)

▶ 150 Calories

▶ 6g Fat

▶ 2g Carbs

▶ 25g Protein

CHAPTER 14

ALCOHOL AND SPIKE LIFE

ALCOHOL BASICS

7 calories per gram—TEF 20%
(Spike Life Goal: Enjoy in Moderation)

Many people want to know if it's ok to consume alcohol with Spike Life. The answer is yes, but it should definitely be in moderation. Alcohol does have 7 calories per gram and I would prefer we eat our calories rather than drink them. Drinking our calories does very little for satiety, and since we have calorie limits, it's best not to waste our calories on things that will not provide us any nutritional benefits. That being said, there are some positives to alcohol.

Positives:

- ▶ Reduces stress
- ▶ 20% TEF
- ▶ Improves insulin sensitivity
- ▶ Moderate drinkers live longer than non-drinkers
- ▶ Alcohol calories cannot be stored as fat
- ▶ Organic wines are high in antioxidants

Negatives:

- ▶ High calories
- ▶ Very low satiety
- ▶ Lowers our inhibitions and increases odds of overeating
- ▶ While drinking alcohol, the other calories we consume have a higher probability of being stored as fat

Spike Life Tips on Alcohol and Weight Loss:

- ▶ Drink in moderation daily

- ▶ Don't eat high calorie foods while drinking
- ▶ Avoid sugary drinks
- ▶ Choose organic wines

CHAPTER 15

CALORIES SUMMARY

It's true, you can lose weight regardless of the types of foods you choose, as long as you consume less calories than you burn. Personally, I've lost weight on both low-fat and low-carb diets. The common aspects were that I restricted calories and lost weight, but I unfortunately gained the weight back because I couldn't maintain a diet that eliminated entire food groups.

In a 2-year study of low-fat dieters versus low-carb dieters reported in the August 3, 2010 issue of *Annals of Internal Medicine*, both the low-carb and low-fat groups lost about an equal amount of weight, proving that weight can be lost on either type of diet. However, choosing foods based off the Spike Life Pyramid makes losing weight considerably easier; a true lifestyle change makes keeping it off much more likely.

Moderating carbohydrates and prioritizing proteins is important for weight loss

Simply restricting calories is difficult to maintain if you are not eating the right kinds of foods. Yes, a calorie is a calorie when it comes to energy balance, but certain calories offer us vital weight loss benefits. These are the foods that we prioritize while living the Spike Life. This plan is not a low-carb diet, but there are advantages to limiting carbohydrates.

Benefits to limiting carbohydrate calories and prioritizing protein calories:

▶ Less physical hunger
▶ Carbohydrates are non-essential calories
▶ Keeps blood sugar stable
▶ Less insulin and more glucagon
▶ Higher metabolism through the thermic effect of food
▶ Increase strength and muscle tissue

Physical Hunger

Carbohydrates are digested quickly and do not provide us the level of satiety that protein does with the same number of calories.

Carbohydrates are non-essential calories

Fats and protein are *essential* to our health—we *need* them. Carbohydrates, while they can provide great energy, are not needed. We can't live without our essential amino acids and fats, but if we were to cease consuming carbohydrates, we could still live a long and healthy life. Fiber is important for weight loss but simple carbohydrates are not.

Carbohydrates affect insulin more than fats and proteins

High carbohydrate meals can cause our blood sugar to skyrocket up and then crash soon after when insulin is released.

You now know from an earlier chapter in this book that insulin is the energy-storing hormone. It sends the glucose in our blood to the liver to be stored as glycogen; if our glycogen stores are full, the remaining is converted to triglycerides and sent back to our bloodstream to be stored as fat. When our blood sugar goes up and then back down, we go through a lopsided energy period. Think about our typical midmorning and afternoon crashes at work or school. This is the proverbial sugar crash; when our blood sugar crashes back down we are hungry again.

When insulin is released too often you can become insulin resistant. Insulin resistance is similar to becoming tolerant to caffeine. If we have too much insulin too often, it just doesn't effect us anymore. Insulin resistance is a part of metabolic syndrome and the beginning of diabetes and other health problems, like cardiovascular disease.

In contrast, a meal high in protein and natural fats does not affect our insulin the way carbohydrates do. Studies have shown that by combining proteins with carbohydrates lowers the impact of carbohydrates on our blood glucose and insulin.

Action Plan for Success

▸ Use the Spike Life Food Pyramid to plan meals
▸ Create a new positive connection with food by being in control and enjoying them

Food needs to be enjoyed

What I have come to learn is that no food is inherently all bad, but long-term success much more likely when we are living a lifestyle where healthy foods make up the majority of our daily calories. Choosing healthy and natural foods full of essential protein, fats, and nutrients, will allow us to eat fewer calories while satisfying our nutritional needs and curbing hunger.

While there's a time to eat clean, there is also a time to indulge. During my six calorie deficit days, I limit trans fats and sugar, but they still have their place in the Spike Life. Enjoying a piece of birthday cake or having the donut you always crave plays a role in this lifestyle. While it may not provide us with a health benefit, it does provide us with an emotional benefit. Could you imagine if I told you that you could be thin but you could never have a bowl of ice cream again, or you could never eat pizza again?

Would you want that life? Is it worth being thin if we have to deprive ourselves of all of the amazingly delicious foods that we love?

For me the answer is a resounding no, I couldn't live that restricted life. Food isn't just an energy source, it is meant to be enjoyed and celebrated. A life without the foods I love isn't worth being thin because I'd still be miserable.

SPIKE LIFE'S BEST OF THE BEST

The following is a list of the best food sources for healthy fats, carbs, and proteins.

BEST FOODS FOR FATS	BEST FOODS FOR CARBS	BEST FOODS FOR PROTEIN
Coconut Oil	Vegetables	Grass-Fed Beef
Avocados	Fruits	Lean Red Meats
Olives Oil	Steel-Cut Oats	Poultry
Flaxseeds	Whole Grains	Fish
Nuts	Legumes	Milk
Eggs	Quinoa	Pasture Raised Meats

SPIKE LIFE FOOD LIST

FOODS TO EAT:	FOODS TO AVOID:
Grass-fed beef	Processed foods
Fish	Trans-fats
Poultry	Snack cakes
Other lean meat	Cookies
Vegetables	Fast-foods
High fiber foods	Sugar
Beans and legumes	White bread
Nuts	White pasta
Eggs	Vegetable oil
Milk	Hydrogenated oils
Reduced fat cheese	Margarine
Fruits	Butter
Oats	Shortening
Whole grains	High sugar cereals
Bran	High fructose corn syrup
Quinoa	Sugary beverages
Olive oil	Soda
Coconut oil	Juice
Coconut flour	Cream latte's
Organic honey	Ice cream
Agave	Frozen meals
Avocados	
Sweet potatoes	

CHAPTER 16

SPIKE LIFE WEIGHT LOSS PLAN

The first step to developing your personal Spike Life weight loss plan is to determine the appropriate calorie targets. The chart below will give you a calorie range which can be used to plan the 6 days of calorie reduction and a Spike Day calorie target for your one day of Spiking.

SPIKE LIFE CALORIE TARGETS					
MEN			**WOMEN**		
Body Weight	Calorie Range	Spike day Calories	Body Weight	Calorie Range	Spike day Calories
170lbs	1400-1900	3800	20lbs	1200-1300	2600
180lbs	1440-1950	3900	130lbs	1200-1350	2700
190lbs	1500-2000	4000	140lbs	1200-1400	2800
200lbs	1550-2050	4100	150lbs	1200-1450	2900
210lbs	1600-2100	4200	160lbs	1200-1500	3000
220lbs	1650-2150	4300	170lbs	1200-1550	3100
230lbs	1700-2200	4400	180lbs	1200-1600	3200
240lbs	1750-2250	4500	190lbs	1200-1650	3300
250lbs	1800-2300	4600	200lbs	1200-1700	3400
260lbs	1850-2350	4700	210lbs	1225-1725	3500
270lbs	1900-2400	4800	220lbs	1250-1750	3500
280lbs	1950-2450	4900	230lbs	1300-1800	3500
290lbs	2000-2500	5000	240lbs	1325-1825	3500
300lbs	2050-2550	5000	250lbs	1350-1850	3500
310lbs	2100-2600	5000	260lbs	1400-1900	3500
320bs	2150-2650	5000	270lbs	1425-1925	3500
330lbs	2200-2700	5000	280lbs	1450-1950	3500
340lbs	2250-2750	5000	290lbs	1500-2000	3500
350+lbs	2300-2800	5000	300+lbs	1550-2050	3500

GRAMS PER DAILY CALORIE GOAL			
Calories	**Fat Grams**	**Carbs Grams**	**Protein Grams**
1200	44	99	102
1300	48	107	110
1400	51	116	119
1500	55	124	128
1600	59	132	136
1700	62	140	145
1800	66	149	153
1900	70	157	162
2000	73	165	170

Use this chart as a guide for your daily meal plan.

Calories X 34% / 4 = Protein Grams
Calories X 33% / 4 = Carbohydrate Grams
Calories X 33% / 9 = Fat Grams

Find your Calorie Range

While calories are the most important factor, you can lose weight quicker and with less hunger if you follow a balanced diet. Spike Life promotes a healthy balanced diet that is high in protein, fiber, and natural unprocessed foods.

Percent of daily calories I recommend:

34% proteins—33% carbohydrates—33% Dietary Fat

(Another important goal is to get 30-50 grams of fiber daily. Fiber with every meal will help to stabilize blood sugar and control our hunger.)

Spike Life Daily Meal Plan

Studies have shown that meal frequency is irrelevant to our metabolism. So there is no added benefit to eating six small meals a day. However, people tend to be less hungry and have lower blood glucose levels with three meals a day versus six.

Meal Plan Goals:

▶ Stay within your calorie range
▶ Eat when you are hungry
▶ Never go to bed hungry
▶ Log your calories in a journal
▶ Avoid processed foods
▶ Drink water between meals
▶ Plan your meals ahead of time

EXAMPLE OF CALORIE GOALS FOR A WEEK LIVING THE SPIKE LIFE						
Sunday	**Monday**	**Tuesday**	**Wednesday**	**Thursday**	**Friday**	**Saturday**
High Range	Low Range	High Range	Low Range	High Range	Low Range	SPIKE DAY

Daily you can choose to eat within the range any way you want, this is just an example. My rule is if you are more hungry one day, then eat at the high end; if you're not as hungry, eat in the low end. Just make sure to spike once a week.

Become a label reader

When you go grocery shopping check the food labels. Some choices for the same foods offer you more protein and fiber than others. Also, avoid foods with added sugars and hydrogenated oils or trans fats.

Easy way to plan meals & snacks:

- ▶ 7-10 grams of protein per 100 calories
- ▶ 2-3 grams of fiber per 100 calories
- ▶ 7-10 grams of carbohydrates
- ▶ 3-4 grams of dietary fat per 100 calories

EXAMPLE OF SPIKE LIFE DAILY MEAL PLAN: 1500-2000 CALORIE RANGE

MEAL	CALORIES	MY MEAL TIPS
Breakfast	200-300 calories	High protein and fiber and less carbs
Lunch	300-500 calories	Balance of carbs, proteins, and fat
Dinner	500-900 calories	Best time to consume carbohydrates
Snacks	100-200 calories	High protein and fiber when you are hungry

I'm a "nighttime eater," meaning I eat most of my carbohydrates and calories in the evening. This is also called calorie back-loading. Personally, I found many benefits to eating most of my calories at night. It fits my lifestyle, where I'm busy all day long and I really enjoy eating a large dinner and nighttime snack. There may also be additional fat-burning benefits from my calorie back-loading. This is the way I've chosen to eat for the past couple of years, and since then, I have gotten to my leanest point ever for my body.

The benefits of calorie back-loading:

- ▶ I'm the hungriest in the evening and I have more calories available.
- ▶ I have time to prepare a healthy meal.
- ▶ It's easier for me to eat smaller meals in the morning and afternoon and I enjoy eating a large dinner.
- ▶ Back-loading calories may burn more body fat.

Our body is highly insulin sensitive first thing in the morning following a night of fasting, so by keeping my blood sugar balanced I'm keeping insulin low during the day. Then my body will release more of the fat-burning hormone, glucagon.

When we consume a high amount of carbohydrates after fasting, like breakfast, we cause our blood glucose levels to increase quickly. This results in a large insulin response. Insulin then causes our blood glucose to drop, and when that happens, we are hungry yet again. One of the goals of Spike life is to keep our blood sugar stable to lessen the impact of insulin. Having a breakfast high in protein and fiber gives our metabolism an early morning boost and reduces hunger by providing us stable energy for hours. By back-loading carbohydrates in the evening we provide our brain the glucose it needs while we sleep and we allow our body to restore some of the glycogen we burned up during the day.

This is the way I do it. You should eat the way you like. While back-loading may provide a weight loss benefit, what truly matters is overall calories and not feeling hungry and miserable.

SPIKE LIFE HEALTHY DAILY MEAL CHOICES:

BREAKFAST	LUNCH	DINNER
Scrambled Eggs	Grilled Chicken	Breaded Chicken
Protein Shake	Turkey Sandwich	Homemade Pizza
Breakfast Wrap	Center-Cut Steak	Chicken Tacos
Protein Bar	Lean Burger	Pasta with Chicken
Fruit Protein Smoothie	Burrito Bowl	Baked Potatoes

Snacks

While I may plan my meals, I don't really plan my snacks. I have snacks ready for when I need them, but if I'm not hungry I save those extra calories for later when I might be hungry. My snacks are low in calories, usually around 100 calories, but I choose snacks that are high in protein and/or fiber. The role my snacks play is to satisfy my hunger and provide a bridge to my next meal.

My favorite snacks

- Beef Jerky
- Reduced Fat Cheese Sticks
- Raw Veggies
- Fruit
- Peanut Butter (mixed with protein powder)
- Greek Yogurt
- 100-Calorie Low-Carb Protein Shakes

Protein Power Snacks

- Peanut Butter Fudge

- ▶ Protein Power Ice Cream
- ▶ Protein Power Cake Batter Bowls

CHAPTER 17

CUSTOMIZING YOUR SPIKE LIFE PLAN

In creating our individual meal plans, we will choose foods that are high in protein and fiber for each and every meal. High protein and fiber foods almost always fall into the prioritize category. These need to become the staples of our diets, and our number one priority. While the Spike Life plan is not a low-carb or low-fat diet, I would call it a high protein and fiber plan. Since I recommend about one-third of our daily calories to come from fats, carbs, and proteins, it's a very balanced eating plan. With Spike Life we eat all kinds of foods; nothing is taboo or eliminated.

Let's go over the facts about calories and weight loss

1.   What truly matters is overall calories in versus calories out
2.   Meal frequency is insignificant for metabolism
3.   One, three, or six meals a day has the same effect on metabolism
4.   Eating at night does not make you fat
5.   You can choose when you have your largest meal
6.   Foods high in protein and fiber provide the most satiety
7.   It is important to keep our blood sugar stable for fat burning
8.   We need to provide our body with essential nutrients
9.   Seven days of caloric restriction reduces leptin levels
10. Spike Day increases leptin levels and spikes metabolism

Knowing the facts, you are able to customize the Spike Life to fit your lifestyle. If you love eating a large breakfast, you can do that. If you prefer to eat fewer calories during the day because you're busy at work and come home to a large dinner, you can do that too. The most important factors are staying within your calorie range and not constantly feeling hungry.

Plan your meals around the way you like to eat

▸ Are you a nighttime eater?
▸ Do you like to eat a large breakfast?
▸ Do you like eating six small meals a day?
▸ Or do you prefer three larger meals?
▸ Do you like to eat little throughout the day and have a large dinner?

FIND YOUR EATING STYLE

"The Nighttime Eater"

This is me to a T; I have always preferred eating at night. I'm usually not very hungry in the morning, and during the day when I'm busy working, I often forget to eat. Then when I come home from work I'm ready for a large meal. When I used to believe that I had to have six small meals and eat every 2-3 hours for my metabolism. I would often have to force myself to eat something when I wasn't hungry. This made it difficult for me to stay within my calorie range because I would have used up 80% of my daily calories by the time I returned home from work. Even though I had plenty of calories earlier in the day, I was still very hungry in the evening. A small meal at night just wouldn't cut it and I would often overeat.

If this sounds like you then you should plan your daily meals like I do. Have fewer calories for breakfast and lunch, and save the majority of your calories for dinner and a bedtime snack.

"The Breakfast Lover"

If you wake up in the morning ravenous and ready to devour anything it sight, then you are what I call a "Breakfast Lover." If you stay within your calorie range for the full day, then you can have your large breakfast and still lose weight.

Just remember that after a night of fasting, your body is very insulin sensitive, so it's best not to have a high carbohydrate breakfast. Instead, you should combine fiber rich foods like whole grains and vegetables, and also add protein to your breakfast. I love pancakes, but pancakes with syrup will have a high impact on your blood sugar. I mix in fiber powder to my pancake mix, and then blend rolled oats with water in my blender and add that to my mix as well. On top of my pancakes I use sugar-free syrup or agave nectar to keep the calories and sugar content down. On the side I will have fruit and low-fat turkey sausages for my protein.

Having a large breakfast makes it extremely important that you track your daily calories. By journaling you will know how many calories you have left to spread over the rest of your day's meals.

"The Grazer"

If you prefer to eat several small meals all day long instead of a few large ones, you are a "Grazer." Contrary to popular belief, it can be more difficult to keep your blood sugar stable and insulin low by grazing. The reasons are because most of us snack on processed high carbohydrate foods. To graze successfully you need to make sure that, at each snack, you have one serving of Spike Life Priority Foods to help keep your blood sugar stable.

An easy way to track your calories is divide your daily calorie goal by six and then plan your six equal meals accordingly. Grazers should pre-plan their meals and carry food with them. That way they won't be tempted by poor food choices when hunger strikes. I recommend having a cooler in the car or at work, and then always keeping it stocked with snacks that are both healthy and enjoyable.

"Eat Like Grandma and Grandpa"

Our grandparents grew up with the mantra "three square meals a day." In some ways this is the ideal way to eat if you don't already have a preferred way of eating. In the study that proved eating six meals a day had no metabolic benefits, they tested subjects consuming 1, 3, and 6 meals. While they each had the same metabolic effect, the only difference was that at 3 meals a day, subjects were less hungry and their blood sugar was the most stable.

This might be the easiest way to track your calories as you can just take your calorie goal and divide it by three. If you are over or under calories on one meal you can adjust the others. Once again, it is important that at each meal, you have protein and fiber from the Spike Life Priority Food List."Intermittent Fasting"

Believe it or not, you can actually lose weight if you save your calories from the day and eat them all in the evening. I know this goes against everything we've been told in the past, but it's true. Like I've said many times in this book, what truly matters for weight loss are calories for 24 hours and energy balance for several days. If your calorie goal is 1,500 calories and you fast all day long, and then eat 1,500 at one meal in the evening, you will lose weight. It's the Law of Thermodynamics. I have personally tried this approach, and while I believe it can be effective, it just didn't work for me because I needed to eat something during the day.

There are several Spikers who combine intermittent fasting and Spike Days with tremendous success. The key is to still choose the majority of calories in your one meal from the Enjoy and Prioritize foods of the Spike Life Food Pyramid. You wouldn't want to substitute a whole pizza for your large meal. The nutrients you get in the evening will be used by your body the following day when you return to fasting.

SAMPLE DAILY MEAL PLANS
Eat the way you want

	KEY:	
(AM)—Morning Snack	(ANY)—AM or PM	(HF)—High Fiber
(LC)—Low Carb	(PM)—Evening Snack	(RF)—Reduced Fat

"NIGHTTIME EATER"—LARGE DINNER AND AN EVENING SNACK
1,200-1,500 CALORIE RANGE

MEAL	CALORIES	MEAL
Breakfast	200-300	Scrambled Eggs with Turkey Sausage
Lunch	200-300	Grilled Chicken with Broccoli & Carrots
Dinner	500-700	Lean Turkey Burger with (LC) Bun & Potato
Snacks	100-200	(PM)—Frozen Yogurt with Strawberries

"BREAKFAST LOVER"—LARGE BREAKFAST AND SMALLER LUNCH
1,200-1,500 CALORIE RANGE

MEAL	CALORIES	MEAL
Breakfast	400-600	Oatmeal Pancakes with Sausage & Fruit
Lunch	200-300	Turkey Sandwich with (LC) Bread & Veggies
Dinner	300-500	Chicken & Pasta with Veggies
Snacks	100-200	(ANY)—Fruit & (RF) cheese stick

"THE GRAZER"—THREE EQUAL MEALS AND SNACKS
1,200-1,500 CALORIE RANGE

MEAL	CALORIES	MEAL
Breakfast	200-300	Egg Omelet with Veggies
Lunch	200-300	Peanut Butter Wrap on (LC) Tortilla
Dinner	200-300	Chicken Quesadilla on (LC) Tortilla
Snacks	200-300	Fruit Smoothie—Protein Bar—Veggies

"GRANDMA & GRANDPA"—THREE LARGE MEALS AND ONE SNACK IF HUNGRY
1,200-1,500 CALORIE RANGE

MEAL	CALORIES	MEAL
Breakfast	300-500	(HF) Oatmeal with Berries
Lunch	300-500	Turkey Avocado Wrap on (LC) Tortilla
Dinner	300-500	Grilled Salmon with Potatoes & Veggies
Snacks	100-200	Beef Jerky

"INTERMITTENT FASTING"—ONE HUGE MEAL (DINNER & SNACK)
1,200-1,500 CALORIE RANGE

MEAL	CALORIES	MEAL
Breakfast	0	Fast
Lunch	0	Fast
Dinner	700-900	Homemade Chicken Pizza with Fruit & Veggies
Snacks	400-600	Protein Shake & Lean Steak

Tips to remember when meal planning

- Log your calories
- 7-10 grams of protein per 100 calories
- 7-10 grams of carbohydrates per 100 calories
- 3-4 grams of fat per 100 calories
- 2-3 grams of fiber per 100 calories
- Drink water between meals
- Supplement with fiber and protein powder if needed
- Snack on raw veggies between meals
- You don't have to stick with one eating style

PART V

EXERCISE AND SPIKE LIFE

CHAPTER 18

EFFICIENT & EFFECTIVE EXERCISE

The great thing about exercise is that everything works. We move and we burn calories. We lift weights and we get stronger. One of the most important aspects for success is finding a type of exercise that you really enjoy. If you enjoy it, you'll stick to it. While all types of exercise help us lose weight, I prefer short and intense workouts that benefit my goals in just about an hour of week. A big secret of mine is that I don't love to exercise and if I had to spend hours a day doing it, I would eventually quit. This is why I use my diet plan to lose weight and time efficient exercise to improve my health.

Exercise should be part of your new healthy lifestyle

My beliefs about exercise differ from most other personal trainers. I do not exercise to lose weight—yes, I said it. I do not exercise to lose weight! What I mean is the purpose of exercising for me isn't to burn a high amount of calories. I exercise to progressively become stronger, build muscle, and increase cardiovascular endurance. I know exercise; the muscles I build help me to maintain my weight loss and live a healthier life.

There was an article in *Time* magazine that created a quite a stir in the fitness community. You may have seen it; the title of the article was *Why Exercise Won't Make You Thin*. The point of the article was that many people reward themselves after an intense aerobic session with food. The mindset is: I deserve it, or I burned 500 calories, so now I can eat 500 calories. The problem is that it's much easier to eat 500 calories than burn 500 calories. If you go to your local coffee shop and order a latte and bran muffin, you just ate the equivalent of an hour of intense exercise. It's hard to correctly balance the calories you burn and the calories you consume.

In the past I've personally done the exercise path to weight loss. I made sure I exercised an hour every day. By exercising and hour a day I lost weight. The problem was I couldn't keep up with an hour of exercise every single day, and as my workouts became less frequent, I stopped losing weight. If I ever stopped exercising because of injury or I was bored of it, I would regain all the weight that I lost and sometimes more.

Dieting and exercise actually have a negative impact on metabolism, and you know that metabolism is the most important factor to keeping weight off. Most people follow a diet and exercise regime to lose weight, but the vast majority of people who lose weight do eventually gain it back.

As someone who struggled with obesity, I agree with the article, I do believe that "exercise won't make you thin." But as someone who has now lost over 100 pounds and maintained it for several years, I believe exercise is very important to our health and does play an important role in losing weight and keeping it off. Exercise is impor-

Spike Life

tant to living the Spike Life, but you need to find a type of exercise you enjoy doing.

CHAPTER 19

STRENGTH TRAINING

Building muscle through strength training is the best type of exercise to increase metabolism and burn body fat.

TYPES OF STRENGTH TRAINING
Free Weights, Strength Machines, Resistance Bands and Bodyweight Exercises

Strength training can be done a number of ways. While free weights have some benefits by working stabilizer muscles, all types of strength equipment can be effective. Ultimately, building strength is about creating resistance. Machines, bands, bodyweight, and free weights all create resistance for your muscles.

Free Weights
Free weights are great for building muscle, and they allow for a free range of motion. You are not locked into the fixed movement of a machine.

Strength Machines
Strength machines are easy to use and great for beginners. They are safer than free weights because you don't have heavy weights hanging over you. You can also adjust the weight easily.

Resistance Bands
Resistance bands offer a unique exercise experience. As you go through the range of motion, the resistance becomes greater and greater as the bands stretch.

Bodyweight Exercise
The best thing about bodyweight exercises is they can be done anywhere. You can do them at home or in a hotel room. The most common bodyweight exercise is pushups.

Spike Life workouts can be done with most types of equipment, and some of our workouts use them all. When choosing for yourself, it's best to do what you feel comfortable doing. It's OK to skip the free weights and exercise only on machines because you will still become stronger. However, I recommend that you give them a try when feel more comfortable.

Building Muscle

Before I go on about how we will build muscle living the Spike Life, I have to address one of the most common misconceptions about strength training. *Ladies, if you lift weights, you will not become big and "bulky" like us guys do.* This is Diet Myth #8. Muscle tissue is very lean and dense compared to body fat. Having muscle makes us actually look smaller and leaner. Men also have more testosterone, the hormone that allows us to build larger muscles. Muscle and testosterone is the main reason men can typically lose weight quicker and easier than women. Increasing muscle mass also increases our metabolism. This is why strength training is my exercise of choice. It's the only way to burn calories while working out and also burn more calories while at rest. The good news is this benefit works for both men and women.

I personally don't include standard aerobic cardio into my exercise routine. I didn't when I lost 100 lbs and I still don't today. For me, it's boring, tedious, and it was unnecessary for me to reach my goals. I would never tell anyone not to do aerobics if they enjoy it. What I'm saying is, unlike popular opinion, you don't have to do cardio in order to lose weight and be fit.

Lifting Weights Can Be Cardiovascular Exercise

It is important to exercise your heart, along with your other muscles. The way I do this is by adding a cardiovascular aspect to my strength workouts by doing circuit style training. Circuit training means there is little to no rest during periods of your workout. This trick also allows me to build strength and increase my cardiovascular endurance with each and every workout.

Strength Training is a Spike Life Priority

When I tell people that I personally only exercise an hour a week, they have a hard time believing me, but it's true. I'm telling you that you can also reach your goals in as little as an hour a week if you do it the right way.

The most effective and time efficient way to exercise and get results is strength training. Lifting weights not only burns calories while you're doing it, like cardio exercise, but it also increases your metabolism after you have finished exercising.

Training Different Muscle Groups

Most people don't have to worry about doing dozens of different exercises to hit every muscle group. I prioritize compound movements. These exercises hit multiple body parts; because of this, we don't have to worry about the extra isolation exercises that only work one muscle group and waste time. An example of a compound exercise is a bench or chest press. This movement works your chest, shoulder, and triceps muscles. An example of an isolation exercise would be a dumbbell curl, since it only works your biceps muscles.

I split my body into three groups to maximize my workouts
- ▶ Upper Body
- ▶ Lower Body
- ▶ Core

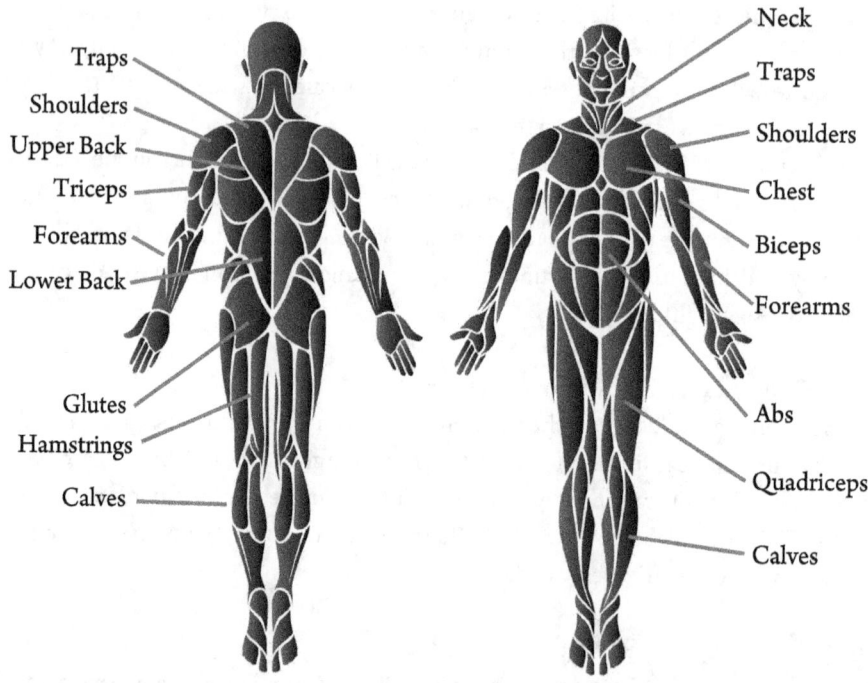

MUSCLE GROUPS		
UPPER BODY	**LOWER BODY**	**CORE**
Neck	Quadriceps	Lower Abs
Traps	Hamstrings	Upper Abs
Chest	Glutes	Obliques
Triceps	Calves	Lower Back
Biceps	Hip Flexors	Upper Back

UPPER BODY EXERCISES

Upper Body Push Exercises	Upper Body Pull Exercises
Bench Press	Dumbbell Row
Dumbbell Press	Compound Back Row
Machine Chest Press	Lat Pull-Down
Push-Ups	Pull-Ups

Push exercises work: chest, front shoulders, and triceps
Pull exercises work: upper and lower back, rear shoulders, traps, and biceps

LOWER BODY EXERCISE

LOWER BODY PUSH EXERCISES	LOWER BODY PULL EXERCISES
Squats	Straight Leg Deadlifts
Leg Press	Leg Curls
Lunges	Deep Squats
Leg Extensions	Reverse Lunges

Push exercises work: quadriceps and calves
Pull exercises work: hamstrings and Gluteus Maximus (butt)

CORE EXERCISES

LOWER ABS	UPPER ABS	OBLIQUE	LOWER BACK
Knee Raises	Sit-Ups	Twist Crunch	Back Extensions
Leg Raises	Crunches	Broom Twist	Planks
Jack Knife	Cable Crunch	Side Jackknife	Deadlifts
Reverse Crunch	Decline Sit-Ups	Side Bend	Good Mornings

Core exercises work: lower abs, upper abs, oblique muscles, and lower back

SPIKE LIFE TIP

Rectus Abdominus is actually one large muscle but different movements put the focus on either the lower or upper parts of the abdominal muscle. I perform different exercises to accentuate development in both my upper and lower abs. Pulling your legs to your body triggers your lower abs and hip flexors. While crunching your upper body down to your core, like a sit-up, triggers your upper abdominal region. Obliques are the muscles on our sides underneath the preverbal "love handles." In order to build a great six-pack you need work all aspects of your core, including your lower back, for muscle balance and stability. I train my abdominals the same way I train every other muscle, with resistance to reach the muscle failure point in the 6-12 rep range. In the past I would do thousands of crunches with nothing to show for it. But once I started using resistance, so I could only complete about a dozen reps before muscle failure, my six-pack started to appear. Since our body loves to store body fat in our core, no matter how strong your abs are, you won't see a thing until diet is under control and you burn fat from that area. If you are overweight you should still do core exercises because your six-pack will be there waiting for you when the fat has been melted away.

CHAPTER 20

CARDIO EXERCISE

While I prefer strength training to cardio exercise because of the additional post exercise benefits of strength training, cardio is still a great way to burn calories. One advantage cardio exercise has over strength training is you can do it daily. When we strength train, we need several days of rest for each muscle group to completely recover. Most cardio exercises don't push our muscles to failure and we can recover much quicker. If we choose to add cardio exercise to our routines, we are able to widen the energy gap and create an even larger deficit of calories and ultimately burn even more body fat. Personally, I rarely do any sort of the traditional cardio exercises. This is simply because I hate cardio! I knew from my past experiences that I would never keep to a cardio routine, so if I lost weight by creating a caloric deficit through cardio exercise, I would gain it right back when I would inevitably quit.

Many people believe that you have to do cardio to drop body fat—Diet Myth #7. That's why one of my goals was to lose weight without cardio, and I did. While I have a personal, major dislike of doing cardio, it is good idea to incorporate at least one cardio session into your weekly routine.

If you love cardio exercise, then feel free to do it as often as you like. You will reap the benefits of increased energy expenditure and lose weight quicker than those like me who choose not to do cardio. Cardio can be done at any time of the day, but some research suggests that early morning pre-breakfast cardio can burn extra body fat for energy. My only concern with exercise in a fasted state is amino acids. My suggestions are to have a small protein shake or BCAAs before you exercise and eat your breakfast soon after you finish your workout.

CARDIO HEART RATE

You reach the cardio heart rate zone when you exercise at 70 to 80 percent of your maximum heart rate. While exercising in the cardio zone, you will be sweating and breathing hard, but you will still able to talk.

Find your Cardio Heart Rate
Men = 220—(age)
Women = 206—(88% of your age)
This is your maximum heart rate (MHR).

Multiply your maximum heart rate by 70% and 80% to find your cardio zone heart rate during aerobic exercise.

Cardio Heart Rate Example:
Leia is 28 years old.

Maximum Heart Rate
28 X 88% = 24.64
206—24.64 = 181.36

181 is Leia's maximum heart rate.

Cardio Heart Rate Zone
181 X 70% = 127
181 X 80% = 145

Leia's Cardio Heart Rate Zone is 127-145 beats per minute.

The American Heart Association suggests that adults under the age of 65 should perform 20 to 30 minutes of cardio several times each week for heart health. With Spike Life we count strength training as a cardio exercise too, because we limit rest in between exercises and our heart rate should be in the cardio zone.

TYPES OF CARDIO TRAINING
High Intensity Training
Medium Intensity Training
Low Intensity Training
High Intensity Interval Training

High Intensity Training (HIT) 80-85% MHR
This type of training is done at around 80-85% of our maximum heart rate. At that point we are out of breath and unable to talk well. High Intensity Training can only be done for very short durations. HIT is very physically demanding, therefore it should only be done when you are already at a good fitness level.

Example:
Sprinting for 5-20 minutes

Medium Intensity Training (MIT) 70-80% MHR
This type of training is done in our cardio zone around 70-80% of our maximum heart rate. At that point we are breathing hard but able to talk. MIT can be done for 20-40 depending on fitness level. This is the typical cardio we do when we take aerobic

classes or use machines at a gym.

Examples:
- Aerobics Class
- Dancing
- Martial Arts
- Bicycling
- Jogging
- Swimming
- Circuit Training
- Cardio Machines

Low Intensity Training (LIT) 40-60% MHR

This type of training is done at around 40-60% of our maximum heart rate. LIT is a great way to start if you are at a beginner training level. At this intensity you can talk easily and still burn fat, because while exercising at a low intensity, you can do it for a longer duration.

Examples:
- Walking
- Yoga
- Cleaning
- Low impact aerobics

High Intensity Interval Training (HIIT) Intervals of 80-85% MHR

This type of training is done in intervals of 80-85% of our maximum heart rate and rest. High Intensity Interval Training (HIIT) is 30-60 second intervals of high intensity cardio, like sprinting, followed by 30-60 seconds of low intensity, like walking or jogging. HIIT should last about 4-15 minutes. This type of exercise is great for burning fat post-exercise with EPOC. EPOC stands for *excess post-exercise oxygen consumption*. This is a fat-burning metabolic boost that lasts for hours after exercise.

Examples:
- Interval Sprinting
- Tabata Training
- Failure & Burn Workouts
- Strength Training
- Interval Cardio
- Spike Life HIIT Workout

HIIT is the Best Cardio for Fat Burning

Each of these types of cardio training has their benefits and they will all help you lose and maintain weight. If I had to choose the best one for fat burning, it would be High Intensity Interval Training (HIIT). HIIT is a hybrid of cardio and strength training. It forces your body to use fast-twitch muscle fibers because of the intensity. Some of types of HIIT can actually build muscle and fatigue you to muscle failure. It is also the best type of cardio to burn body fat post-workout through EPOC. Low Intensity Training (LIT), like walking, is something I recommend you do daily. It's very low impact, yet it increases our energy output.

SPIKE LIFE HOME HIIT WORKOUT

1. WARM-UP: Very Important

EXERCISE	TIME	REST (WALK IN PLACE)
Jumping Jacks	30 seconds	30 seconds
High Knees	30 seconds	30 seconds
Wall Push-Ups	30 seconds	30 seconds

2. REST AN EXTRA MINUTE AND THEN BEGIN

3. SPIKE LIFE HIGH INTENSITY INTERVAL TRAINING: REPEAT 2-3 TIMES

EXERCISE	TIME	REST
Push-Ups	40 seconds	30 seconds
High Knees	40 seconds	30 seconds
Burpees	40 seconds	30 seconds
Jump Squats	40 seconds	30 seconds
Jumping Jacks	40 seconds	30 seconds

The Spike Life Home HIIT workout takes between 10-20 minutes, based on the number of repetitions you complete. Depending on your exercise levels, you may want to just complete one full round or take a longer rest period between exercises. It's better to start out slow and work your way up. You can find descriptions and videos of these exercises at spikelifebook.com

The Best Exercise in the World

Ultimately, the best overall type of exercise isn't the one that burns the most calories, it's the one that you enjoy and will stick to. Don't try fitting round pegs into square holes. In other words, don't force yourself to do an exercise if you despise it. You will end up dreading working out and eventually you will quit. Instead, I recommend trying a bunch of different exercises in the beginning, from gym group classes to workout DVDs. Find something you truly enjoy and do that for a while. When you feel yourself getting bored with it, try something new. Focus on progression with each workout and you will be successful.

Calories Burned Exercising

Our immediate reward for exercising is seeing how many calories we burned. It can be a motivation tool when you can visually see the amount of calories you are burning. If you're close to 500 calories, you may exercise a few more minutes to reach that number. Or if you burn 300 calories one day, your goal the next day could be to burn 350 calories. It's immediate gratification for your hard work. While I mentioned before, my purpose of exercise isn't to lose weight; but at the same time, the calories we burn definitely helps if we don't just eat the calories back. I believe that wearing calorie counters is a great idea and tool to keep us motivated. I think they should be used to push us to reach a goal for burning calories, but not as a guide for how much we should eat when the goal is weight loss. Calories burned through exercise are a product of intensity and duration.

INTESITY x DURATION = CALORIES BURNED

The more intensive the workout, the more your body has to work. This way, you burn more calories per minute than lower intensity exercises allow. On the flip side, you can work out much longer at a lower intensity before fatigue makes you quit. There really isn't a right or wrong way, just your way. If you are able to complete intense workouts and you have less time to exercise, then go the high intensity route. If you are a beginner, you can still burn calories at a low intensity by working out longer.

The Fat-Burning Zone

"The Fat-Burning Zone" is Diet Myth #9. While it's true we burn a higher percentage of fat in this zone, we burn more overall calories per minute in higher intensity zones. Expending more calories leads to increased fat burning.

ESTIMATING EXERCISE CALORIES BURNED PER HOUR

It's a motivational tool to know approximately how many calories you are burning with your hard work. These are simple estimates. The more you weigh, the more calories you burn exercising. The low end of the range is for those who weigh around 150 lbs and the high end is 250 lbs. There is a more accurate calories burned calculator at spikelifebook.com

ESTIMATED CALORIES BURNED PER HOUR

EXERCISE	CALORIES BURNED PER HOUR
Aerobics (Medium Intensity)	533-796
Aerobics (Low Intensity)	365-545
Backpacking	511-763
Basketball Game	584-872
Bicycling (LIT)	292-436
Bowling	219-327
Canoeing	256-382
Dancing	219-327
Football	584-872
Golfing (no cart)	314-469
Hiking	438-654
Jumping Rope	861-1,286
Ice Skating	511-763
Racquetball	511-763
Resistance Strength Training	365-545
Rollerblading	548-818
Rowing	438-654
Running, 5 mph	606-905
Running, 8 mph	861-1,286
Skiing, Cross-Country	496-741
Skiing, Downhill	314-469
Softball or Baseball	365-545
Stair Climbing	657-981
Swimming	423-632
Tae Kwon Do	752-1,123
Tai Chi	219-327
Tennis	584-872
Volleyball	292-436
Walking, 2 mph	204-305
Walking, 3.5 mph	314-469
Water Skiing	438-654

CHAPTER 21

STRENGTH WORKOUTS

Fitness is full of irony. I find it funny that losers win and failure equals success.

My workouts, while short in duration, are definitely intense and very effective.

There are two main components of my strength workouts; I call them "Failure & Burn" workouts.

Going to Failure for Success

When we exercise to failure we greatly enhance the muscle building process. You've learned how our body adapts during starvation mode; well, building muscle is also a form of adaptation. I will use a chest bench press as an example; when I am bench pressing, my body is igniting muscle fibers to press the weight up and down from my chest. When I first start lifting the weight, the first few reps are fairly easy; as I continue, my muscles become more fatigued. When I get to the point that I am so fatigued I can no longer complete a full rep, I hit failure. I failed to complete a rep. My body then wants to adapt and become stronger, so the next time I will not fail on that rep. So the following week, when I do that extra rep, I have successfully progressed and became stronger. Of course, I go beyond that completed rep, and fail at the next one. Going to failure with each muscle group is the most efficient way to progress and build muscle, which ultimately leads to greater fat burning due to a higher metabolism.

One-Set Failure Training

In my years of experience lifting weights, the principle of training to failure has been by far the most successful. With Spike Life Workouts, we only focus on one "working set" for each muscle group. The working set is the only set that really matters. This plan is different than most typical workout routines that may have you doing 3, 4, or even 6 sets. This way we can put all of our effort into that one set. You only have to train to failure for one set to get the benefits. When you hit that failure point, you're done and it's time to move on to the next exercise. There is a huge mental advantage to one-set failure training. You don't have to *pace* yourself, and you can put maximum effort into moving as much weight as possible for just one set. Being an ex-football player, I call this mentality "leaving it all on the field."

If you are a beginner to strength training, I highly recommend that you consult with your doctor before following this training principle. It is also a great idea to meet with a personal trainer so they can teach you proper lifting form, so you can avoid injury. For beginners, it is OK to stop just before failure too, especially since your muscles are not used to being trained.

As your muscles become more efficient, they progress less and less. This is when it is a good time to change up your exercises and start incorporating some advanced failure techniques.

> ❗ SPIKE LIFE TIP
> You should always have a trained spotter helping you when you exercise to failure with free weights.

ADVANCED FAILURE TECHNIQUES
Drop Set
Forced Rep
Negative Rep
Rest and Go
Isometric Hold

Drop Set

A drop set is when you lift as much as you can with a heavy weight and immediately drop the weight down, and then complete more reps with a lower weight. This is done easily using a strength training machine that uses plates and pins for weight resistance. For example: if you are doing a machine chest press, when you get to the point when you can't complete another rep, you would set the weight back, move the pin to the spot that is 20-50 pounds less, and do a few more reps.

Forced Rep

Forced reps are done with a training partner or a spotter. When you get to the point of failure, your partner would assist you in completing an extra rep.

Negative Rep

A negative rep is also done using a spotter. Much like a forced rep, when you get to the point of failure, you keep going. This time you focus on the negative portion of the exercise at a slow pace. I usually do a count of three to five. Your partner then helps you bring the weight back through the positive portion of the lift.

Rest and Go

Rest and go is when you reach failure on your move and then set the weight back and rest for 10-20 seconds. After your rest, you try and complete another rep. Rest and go should also be done with a spotter if you are doing free weights.

Isometric Hold

Isometric holds are great at the end of a set. "Isometric" refers to the muscle contraction. When I flex my bicep and ask, "Is the beach that way?", I'm doing an isometric hold. While it would be difficult to build muscle by simply flexing, it can be that little extra bonus at the end of the set that helps you become stronger. To perform an isometric hold, you simply hold the last rep in about the halfway point of a movement, and flex or contract the muscle you are working. You hold this pose for three to five seconds and then set the weight back. Isometric holds are best done with strength machines. If you attempt to do these with free weights, make sure you use a spotter.

Feel the Burn!

I'm sure you have heard it before: "Feel the burn!" Well, Spike Life workouts will make you feel the burn. The burn is actually a buildup of lactic acid in your muscles. While many people try to avoid the burn, and for a long time the "burn" or "pump" was viewed as unnecessary and only served a short-lived visual reward for narcissistic bodybuilders. Research now shows that lactic acid plays a large role in building muscle, and the pump is more valuable than just looking at a mirror. We now know that lactic acid leads to increased growth hormone release. After we finish working out, our body releases a growth hormone to help us recover and rebuild muscle tissue. The amount of growth hormone secreted is largely dependent on the amount of lactic acid that was built up in our muscles. The more burn we feel, the more growth hormone will be released. This leads to greater amounts of lean body mass and a higher level of fat-burning.

The other benefit of the burn is increased blood flow. Amino acids and other nutrients our muscles need are transported through our blood. By increasing the blood flow to our muscle, we kick start the recovery process and provide our muscles the ammo they need to become stronger.

To get the best results we follow up our one-set failure with a circuit-style exercise that I call the "gauntlet." Years ago when I played football, we had a drill that was called the gauntlet. For this drill, the football team would create two lines and we'd leave one poor kid in the middle. The goal of the drill was for the one kid to run his way between the two lines while the other fifty guys would try to knock him on his tail. It was extremely intense. The gauntlet for strength training is also extremely intense. It is what is called a giant set; it combines three different exercises for the same muscle group. The sets are completed one after another without rest. We use lighter weights and try to complete a high amount of reps, 12-15 for each exercise. Once you complete one full set of the three exercises, you do it two more times, without a rest. The gauntlet gives us the pump we need and it is also a tremendous cardiovascular workout. When you're done, you will feel exhausted but you will also know you worked to your peak.

By focusing on one-set failures and the gauntlet, Spike Life workouts are both time efficient and extremely effective. A week worth of workouts takes approximately one hour. This can be done with one workout a week or you can split it up. Some people prefer two half-hour sessions or three twenty-minute sessions. Much like our daily meal plans, you can customize the workout to fit your schedule and do it the way you like. If you are feeling confused about sets, reps, and just how to put together a workout, don't worry. I will walk you through a few sample workouts so you will better understand how to complete a Spike Life workout.

CHAPTER 22

THE ONE-HOUR A WEEK WORKOUT

In this Chapter, I show you three workouts that focus on the main muscle groups: Upper Body, Lower Body, and Core.

Each workout is done using Spike Failure & Burn principles. These workouts are intense and you should definitely talk to your doctor before attempting this or any other exercise routine.

You can do these workouts on different days of the week. I recommend you do at least one of these workouts the day after your Spike Day. "Spiked" workouts are amazing for both strength and endurance.

You can complete all three workouts in the same day instead of splitting them up. I've done this many times in the past when I could only make it to the gym one day a week. Doing them all in one day can be very demanding on your body, so I recommend you just do one set of the Spike Gauntlet per workout and rest five minutes between each workout.

EXAMPLE OF SPLITTING FAILURE & BURN WORKOUTS OVER THE WEEK						
SUNDAY	**MONDAY**	**TUESDAY**	**WEDNESDAY**	**THURSDAY**	**FRIDAY**	**SATURDAY**
Upper Body	*Cardio & Rest*	Lower Body	*Cardio & Rest*	Core	HIIT	SPIKE DAY

Doing all of the Failure & Burn Workouts on One Day
Workout #1 Upper Body 15-20 minutes
Rest 5 Minutes
Workout #2 Lower Body 15-20 Minutes
Rest 5 Minutes
Workout #3 Core   15-20 Minutes

Only complete one set of the Spike Gauntlet for each workout. Drink plenty of water during the workouts. If you choose to do all three body groups on the same day, I recommend you do it the day after spiking for maximum effectiveness.

FAILURE & BURN WORKOUT #1

Muscle Group: Upper Body Duration: 20-30 Minutes
Going to "failure" is key for progression and "burning out" is important for recovery

ORDER	EXERCISE	MUSCLES TRAINED	SET 1	SET 2	SET 3
ONE-SET "FAILURE" EXERCISES (REST 60 SECONDS BETWEEN EXERCISES)					
1	Bench Press	Chest Shoulders Triceps	Warm-up	Warm-up	*
2	Machine Row	Lower Back Biceps Traps	Warm-up	Warm-up	*
3	Shoulder Press	Shoulders Triceps Upper Chest	SKIP	Warm-up	*
4	Lat Pull-Down	Upper Back Biceps Traps	SKIP	Warm-up	*
SPIKE "BURN" GAUNTLET (NO REST - TO FAILURE WITH LIGHTER RESISTANCE)					
5	Push-Ups	Chest Shoulders Triceps	12-20 reps	12-20 reps	12-20 reps
6	Pull-Ups	Back Biceps	12-20 reps	12-20 reps	12-20 reps
7	Bench Dip	Chest Shoulders Triceps	12-20 reps	12-20 reps	12-20 reps
8	Dumbbell Rows	Back Biceps Traps	12-20 reps	12-20 reps	12-20 reps

* 6-9 rep range for advanced lifters and 10-15 for beginners (See trainer tips below)

Trainer Tips:

▶ Talk to your doctor before beginning this or any other exercise program.
▶ Novice weight lifters should begin with resistance machines instead of free weights.
▶ Exercises #1-4 are One-Set Failure exercises.

- ▶ Warm-up with light resistance in the 10-15 rep range.
- ▶ The Set #3: "working set," 6-9 rep range for advanced lifters and 10-15 for beginners.
- ▶ The goal is progression. Each week increase reps or weight.
- ▶ Exercises #5-8 are the Spike Gauntlet.
- ▶ Spike Gauntlet is a circuit-style giant-set without rest.
- ▶ Beginners should begin slowly and **rest** if needed.
- ▶ Begin with one set of the Spike Gauntlet and work your way up to 3 sets.
- ▶ Rep range for the Spike Gauntlet is 12-20 with light resistance.

FAILURE & BURN WORKOUT #2

Muscle Group: Lower Body Duration: 20-30 Minutes
Going to "failure" is key for progression and "burning out" is important for recovery

ORDER	EXERCISE	MUSCLES TRAINED	SET 1	SET 2	SET 3
ONE-SET "FAILURE" EXERCISES (REST 60 SECONDS BETWEEN EXERCISES)					
1	Squat	Quads Hamstrings Glutes	Warm-up	Warm-up	*
2	Leg Curl	Hamstrings Glutes	Warm-up	Warm-up	*
3	Leg Extension	Quads	SKIP	Warm-up	*
4	Calf Raises	Calves	SKIP	Warm-up	*
SPIKE "BURN" GAUNTLET (NO REST - TO FAILURE WITH LIGHTER RESISTANCE)					
5	Lunges	Quads Hamstrings Glutes	30-60 Seconds	30-60 Seconds	30-60 Seconds
6	Jump Squat	Quads Hamstrings Glutes	30-60 Seconds	30-60 Seconds	30-60 Seconds
7	Reverse Lunge	Quads Hamstrings Glutes	30-60 Seconds	30-60 Seconds	30-60 Seconds
8	Treadmill Sprint	Quads Hamstrings Glutes	30-60 Seconds	30-60 Seconds	30-60 Seconds

* 6-9 rep range for advanced lifters and 10-15 for beginners (See trainer tips below)

Trainer Tips:

▶ Talk to your doctor before beginning this or any other exercise program.
▶ Novice weight lifters should begin with resistance machines instead of free weights.
▶ Exercises #1-4 are One-Set Failure exercises.· Warm-up with light

resistance in the 10-15 rep range.

▶ The Set #3: "working set," 6-9 rep range for advanced lifters and 10-15 for beginners.

▶ The goal is progression. Each week increase reps or weight.

▶ Exercises #5-8 is the Spike Gauntlet.

▶ Spike Gauntlet is a circuit-style giant set without rest.

▶ Beginners should begin slowly and rest if needed.

▶ Begin with one set of the Spike Gauntlet and work your way up to 3 sets.

▶ Rep range for the Spike Gauntlet is 12-20 with light resistance.

FAILURE & BURN WORKOUT #3

Muscle Group: "Hard-Core" Duration: 20-30 Minutes
Going to "failure" is key for progression and "burning out" is important for recovery

ORDER	EXERCISE	MUSCLES TRAINED	SET 1	SET 2	SET 3
ONE-SET "FAILURE" EXERCISES (REST 60 SECONDS BETWEEN EXERCISES)					
1	Knee Raises w/ Resistance	Lower Abs Hip Flexors	Warm-up	Warm-up	*
2	Decline Crunch w/ Resistance	Upper Abs	Warm-up	Warm-up	*
3	Side Crunch w/ Resistance	Obliques	Warm-up	Warm-up	*
4	Hyper Extensions	Low Back	Warm-up	Warm-up	*
SPIKE "BURN" GAUNTLET (NO REST - TO FAILURE WITH LIGHTER RESISTANCE)					
5	Plank	Abs Low Back	30-60 Seconds	30-60 Seconds	30-60 Seconds
6	Side Plank	Abs Obliques Low Back	30-60 Seconds	30-60 Seconds	30-60 Seconds
7	Hip Thrust	Abs Low Back	30-60 Seconds	30-60 Seconds	30-60 Seconds
8	Lying Leg Raise	Lower Abs Hip Flexors	30-60 Seconds	30-60 Seconds	30-60 Seconds

* 6-9 rep range for advanced lifters and 10-15 for beginners (See trainer tips below)

TRAINER TIPS:

▶ Talk to your doctor before beginning this or any other exercise program.
▶ Novice weight lifters should begin with resistance machines instead of free weights.
▶ Exercises #1-4 are One-Set Failure exercises.
▶ Warm-up with light resistance in the 10-15 rep range.
▶ The Set #3: "working set," 6-9 rep range for advanced lifters and 10-15 for beginners.

- ▶ The goal is progression. Each week increase reps or weight.
- ▶ Exercises #5-8 is the Spike Gauntlet.
- ▶ Spike Gauntlet is a circuit-style giant set without rest.
- ▶ Beginners should begin slowly and rest if needed..
- ▶ Begin with one set of the Spike Gauntlet and work your way up to 3 sets.
- ▶ Rep range for the Spike Gauntlet is 12-20 with light resistance.

CHAPTER 23
SPIKE LIFE EXERCISE SUMMARY

The goal of losing weight with Spike Life is to do it mostly through diet, and use exercise to support our weight loss. Exercise is extremely important to our overall health, but I want us to stop seeing exercise as a "necessary evil" and instead, see it as something we actually enjoy doing.

Remember, the best exercise in the world is the type of exercise that you think is fun. Combine a fun workout by motivating yourself with progression and results, and you will no longer dread working out. Instead, you will begin to looking forward to it.

I want you to commit to at least one hour a week of exercise and eventually you may *want* to do more. If you already enjoy exercising, you can do it as often as you like, I just recommend taking Spike Day off to give yourself a break and a day to recharge.

Rest and Recovery

When we exercise we are preparing our body to adapt to our environment by building muscle to become stronger. We don't actually build muscle during our workout; we build it while we are at rest and while we sleep. This is why proper recovery is a necessity living the Spike Life. Recovery begins the minute we are finished with our workout; this why it's important to have quick digesting protein, like whey protein, immediately after strength training. I recommend 15-30g for women and 20-40g for men. This quickly fills our blood with the amino acids our body needs to start repairing muscle tissue and kick starts the recovery process.

Muscle Soreness

Everyone knows lifting weights causes muscle soreness. This is a normal part of the recovery process. Delayed Onset Muscle Soreness, DOMS, happens 24-48 hours after you exercise. You are sore because your body is repairing muscle and it doesn't want you to aggravate those muscles while it's repairing them. Having an ample amount of protein in your diet helps quicken recovery and lessen soreness. Muscle soreness is a reason why we break our body down into groups for strength training, because you need to rest the muscles you train several days before they are ready to be worked again. When you split your body groups up, you can strength train efficiently three or four times a week without upsetting the recovery process. Sometimes it takes longer to recover. My rule of thumb is: If a muscle is sore, don't train it. Wait an extra day or two until it's ready. In place of that muscle's workout, you could do a session of cardio or work a different muscle group.

When you are a beginner, it's tough to know if your soreness is normal or an injury. If you are unsure I recommend talking to a Personal Trainer or your doctor to make sure an injury did not occur.

Sleep

It is extremely important to get 7-8 hours of straight sleep every night. Studies have shown that people who sleep less or more usually struggle with losing weight. While we are sleeping, growth hormone peaks and our body has a great opportunity to re-build muscle and burn fat.

You also never want to go to bed hungry. I recommend having casein protein right before you hit the hay. If your body doesn't have amino acids available to rebuild muscle, it will actually attack other muscles to take out the amino acids it needs to rebuild another muscle. This leads to a decline in lean body mass and metabolism. Casein protein before bed is a naturally time released protein that will provide your body hours of amino acids while you are in a fasted state. In scientific research, the benefits of casein protein have been recently proven to help us build muscle and save muscle wasting while we sleep. A simple and cheap way to get casein protein is to have a glass of milk before bed.

Strength Training Versus Cardio

All exercise is good and valuable. Strength training has a few more long-term weight loss benefits than cardio, so it's my preferred style of exercise. Cardio exercise has more options to try if you get bored easily with one type of workout. You can also do it daily, whereas with strength training you need to allow time for rest and recovery. The ideal way to exercise is to do both; prioritize strength training but mix in cardio on the off-days. If you do them on the same day, I recommend strength training first, then take a short break and have a whey protein drink, and then perform your cardio routine. You need more energy for effective strength training, and cardio can be done with less energy.

Hiring a Personal Trainer

If you have a limited knowledge of workouts, I highly recommend you hire a personal trainer. Certified personal trainers are professionals that will customize workouts for you and teach you proper exercise form to avoid injury. When hiring a trainer, I believe you should look for someone who understands your struggles and who you feel you can confide with when you need support.

Things to ask for when hiring a trainer
- Accreditations
- Work Experience
- Education
- References

- ▸ Rates
- ▸ Liability Insurance
- ▸ If they provide equipment for in-home training
- ▸ How they can help you

Hiring a personal trainer isn't cheap, so make sure you get your money's worth. If you don't think the relationship is working well, tell your trainer how you feel and don't feel bad about looking for a new one.

Joining a Gym

I know from past experience that it can be extremely difficult to have efficient workouts at home. A gym membership can be as cheap as $1 a day and it is very much worth it. You will have access to all types of equipment and an escape to get away and focus on your workout without distractions at home.

Home Exercise

Exercising at home can be very effective with the right equipment. Strength training is just resistant training. Resistance can come from free weights, machines, bands, and even just your bodyweight. Home exercise equipment ranges from less expensive resistance bands and dumbbells to expensive full home gyms. If you can't afford expensive equipment, or you're not able to get a full workout, then I recommend a gym membership where you have many more options to choose from.

> **SPIKE LIFE TIP**
> I have both a gym membership and home exercise equipment, so I have the option to do both depending on my free time and the workout. I find most of my home exercise equipment cheap at garage sales, local online sales listings sites, and online auction sites. After the New Year I typically find a flood of listings for hardly used exercise equipment for less than half the cost of new.

MY FINAL MESSAGE

There are few goals in life that are more amazing to accomplish than losing weight forever. Our environment makes gaining weight easy and our nature makes losing it difficult. I want you to remember that it's not your fault if you are overweight; it's only natural considering the way our bodies are hard-wired and the perfect storm of obesity that surrounds us.

Be Motivated!

Despite that, you can, without a doubt, change your situation. With motivation and commitment, anything is possible. If you can dream it, you can do it! I want you to take on this challenge with complete confidence and truly enjoy each and every day of your journey to freedom from obesity. The knowledge in this book will be your guide, making your expedition far less complicated and the successful arrival to your goals much more likely.

Stay in Control

One major advantage Spiking gives you is control. You are the Master of Your Universe and you have the power to create the life and the body that you really want to have. Stay in control over your food. Spikers don't fall off the wagon; they jump off when they choose to. If you do slip up, don't worry about it and move on. The guilt you feel is far more damaging than the extra calories.

Log Your Calories

I can't stress enough that it is extremely important to log your daily calories. This will show you where you are doing well and what might need refining. Remember, people who track calories in journals lose twice as much as those who don't. This is a way to show your commitment and also your control over living a healthy life.

Be Patient

Remember to stay patient. We all wish just reading this book would immediately make us lose weight—and it does! Sorry, not really, that wasn't nice of me, but you know it takes time and effort. You will lose weight if you stay patient and stick to it. There will be weeks with great weight loss and others without. That really doesn't matter. This is a long-term lifestyle and not a quick-fix. Living the Spike Life creates a weekly caloric deficit, so in the long run you will indeed lose weight. After all, it's the law.

Have a Positive Relationship with Food

Many of us who struggle with weight have a negative relationship with food. It's like any abusive relationship. We love it and we hate it. We break up with it and we struggle to get it out of our hearts and our minds but it always comes back. Food can make us happy in the moment and break our hearts minutes later. We feel jealousy when we can't have it and we see it with someone else. Then, even when we know it's bad for us, we still let it back into our lives. Knowing that food is more than just calories and energy and realizing the fact that we have an emotional and physical connection to it gives us power. We have to accept that we can't live without our favorite foods, because it's true love that will never simply go away. Finding a way to lose weight without giving up the foods we love is the key to long-term success. I found that the amazing truth is we can change this abusive relationship into one that can actually benefit us.

In the battle of obesity, Spike Life turns those foods from our weight loss enemies to comrades on our side. By spiking they become strategically placed weapons that help us destroy body fat once and for all, so we can win our freedom from obesity.

I want you to have a positive relationship with food like other Spikers. This is done by taking control and truly understanding how calories and our bodies are connected.

Spike Day is Retribution!

Fully enjoy your Spike Day. It's like laughing in the face of dieting, the dieting that has caused us years of frustration and heartache. Spike Days are our retribution for the years of pain caused from struggling with our weight and every failed diet. Remember that even with a day of calorie surplus, you will be in a weekly caloric deficit, which will facilitate your weight loss. Spike Days keep your metabolism honest and you mentally refreshed and motivated.

Take this Opportunity to Redefine Yourself

Skinny people have no idea how amazing it feels to overcome this lifelong obstacle. You will have the rare opportunity to redefine yourself and become the person you want to be! When you have this new confidence in your appearance, it will allow you to show your true self to the people around you. I know this from my experience when I was overweight. I would try and hide myself and just blend in so no one would see me, even though at my size, I'm not sure how they could miss me. Now I love talking to people. Instead of hiding amongst the crowd, now I'm like, "Hey look at me!" Losing weight completely changed my life. It improved how I look, act, and feel. I'm physically younger, healthier, and fully enjoying an amazing Spiked Life. Your happiness matters to me. This is why I am sharing this gift with you. I want you to love spiking and live a Spiked Life with me.

God Bless,

Russell Branjord

You can connect with me directly at spike84.com and spikelifebook.com

PART VI

SPIKE LIFE SUPPLEMENT GUIDE

Supplements help a good plan, but they don't make a good plan.

I am often asked about supplements and what one can take to lose weight or build muscle. Regardless of what adds in a magazine may say, the truth is there is nothing we can take to do either. However, I do take supplements, and the ones I take are the ones I recommend. I take supplements to help me progress and *supplement* my healthy eating and exercise plan.

Supplements can help with:
- ▶ Recovery
- ▶ Health
- ▶ Appetite Suppressants
- ▶ Energy
- ▶ Sleep

SPIKE LIFE SUPPLEMENT GUIDE
(These supplements are safe for most healthy adults, but you need to talk to your doctor to make sure they are right for you.)

SUPPLEMENTS FOR DAILY USE
Multivitamin
Taking a multivitamin first thing in the morning with breakfast is a cheap and easy way to defend against any potential vitamin and mineral deficiencies in your diet. It may not be needed, but I do take one. I feel like it's better to safe than sorry.

Usage: One pill daily in the morning. It doesn't need to be an expensive brand.

Vitamin D
Most of us do not get enough Vitamin D in our diet. Deficiencies in Vitamin D can lead to our bodily functions running less than ideal. Also some research has shown that Vitamin D may boost strength and athletic performance.

Usage: 2000 IU per day is a safe dosage, but I know of many people who use considerably higher doses without any negative side effects.

Omega 3—Fish Oil

Maintaining a good omega-3 to omega-6 ratio is extremely important. Most of us we get too much omega-6 and not enough omega-3. Getting our essential fatty acids is vital for our hormone production and overall health.

Usage: Take 2 grams of fish oil high in omega-3s daily with food.

Arginine

Arginine is a semi-essential amino acid. It is a precursor to nitric oxide, which helps widen blood vessels and increase blood flow. It helps our body to create protein and it's been shown to enhance muscle building and tissue wasting.

Usage: Men take 3-5 grams, women take 1-3 grams daily in the morning or pre-workout.

Branched Chain Amino Acids

BCAAs are linked amino acids that aid with intra-set recovery and muscle endurance in the higher rep ranges. I use BCAAs pre-workout and if I am getting hungry between my meals as an appetite suppressant.

Usage: Take 5-10 grams pre-workout or between meals; each gram counts as a protein and four calories in your food log.

Calcium

Calcium increases fat excretion and boosts testosterone in men. If you get enough calcium through your diet, there's no need to take extra from a supplement.

Usage: Take 500-750mg each day if needed to supplement your diet.

Glutamine

Glutamine is the most abundant amino acid in the body, but when we exercise our body may need more of it. Glutamine helps repair our tissues and build muscle by limiting cortisol. It has been used to treat Irritable Bowel Syndrome (IBS).

Usage: Take 5 grams before bed to limit cortisol release overnight.

Glucosamine

I've used glucosamine periodically when my joints are sore and after I had shoulder surgery several years ago. Studies show that glucosamine is a safe and effective supplement for relieving pain and stiffness in joints. You should talk to your doctor when you have joint pain to make sure it is not a serious injury.

Usage: Take 1.5 grams daily.

Melatonin

Sleep is extremely important to living a healthy Spike Life. When we sleep well our body releases growth hormones. With a good night's sleep we are better able to recover from exercise and growth hormones help us burn body fat for energy. Our natural melatonin helps control our sleep cycle. When melatonin is high, we are tired and ready to sleep. I've used melatonin supplements many times in the past when I was struggling to fall asleep. For most adults, melatonin supplements are safe in low doses for both short and long-term use. But you should talk to with your doctor about taking them.

Usage: Take 1-3mg before bed when you feel you need help to fall asleep.

SUPPLEMENTS I USE ON WORKOUT DAYS

Creatine

There are several scientific studies to support its ability to help us exercise more effectively and build lean body mass. Increasing muscle creatine gives our workouts a boost, and with more effective workouts, we are able to build more lean body mass. There are hardly any side effects with creatine and it can be used by both men and women.

Usage: Take 5 grams pre-workout.

Rhodiola

Rhodiola has been shown to improve mental focus and reduce fatigue. It can be helpful pre-workout by increasing your alertness and energy. It can be used as a daily energy supplement.

Usage: Take 200-600mg daily pre-workout or daily in the morning. It can be used by both men and women.

Beta-Alanine

Beta-Alanine is an amino acid that has been shown to boost exercise performance. It is extremely effect for intense exercise like Spike Failure & Burn workouts.

Usage: Men take 4 grams daily if you're following a strength training routine.

PROTEIN SUPPLEMENTS

Whey Protein Powders

Whey protein has the highest biological value of all proteins and it's also absorbed very quickly, making whey ideal for post-workout. Whey is the benchmark for all protein powders, but it's not great as a meal replacement because it's absorbed too quickly and won't provide a break from hunger.

Usage: 20-40g post-workout for men and 15-30g post-workout for women.

Casein Protein Powders

Casein protein is another milk protein that is natural and time released. It's perfect to use as a pre-bedtime snack. It is the opposite of whey and absorbed slowly, making it a poor post-workout option but great as a meal replacement.

Usage: 20-40g for men and 15-30g for women as a meal replacement or pre-bedtime snack.

SUPPLEMENTS THAT CAN AID IN WEIGHT LOSS

Caffeine

Caffeine has been shown to increase energy, suppress appetite, and increase metabolism through thermogenesis.

Usage: Take 100-200mg daily in the morning and before workouts.

Inulin Fiber Powder

Inulin is a tasteless soluble fiber that can decrease hunger and help you lose weight. It mixes easily and can be added to water or other beverages. I also add it to some foods when I need extra fiber during the day.

Usage: Supplement your diet with 5 grams a few times a day between meals.

PART VII

APPENDIX

Spike Life Success Stories
In Their Own Words
Spike Diet Customer Reviews

Charts and Guides
Spike Life Quick Start Guide
BMI
BMR
TDEE
Estimating Weight Loss
Food Fullness Grades
Grocery Shopping List
Lower Calorie Snacks
Blank Food Journal
Blank Exercise Log
Spike Life Tips
A Few of my Favorite Things...
Glossary
References

SPIKE LIFE SUCCESS STORIES

IN THEIR OWN WORDS

From Fat to Fit to Ripped

I remember as a child watching my two uncles posing and flexing their gigantic muscles and I was in complete awe. They both competed in bodybuilding and owned their own gym in the small town where I grew up in central Indiana. I was at a very impressionable age, maybe ten or eleven years old, and knew that I wanted what they had, muscles and veins everywhere. From those early days on, I aspired to be like them. I wanted to be big and lean.

Fast forward ten years to my early 20s. I was hitting the gym hard and getting stronger weekly. I loved my time in the gym and was making great progress. I managed to hit my lifelong goal, 300 lbs on the bench press and I thought I was really figuring things out. I even started having people in the gym ask me for advice. At this time my image in the mirror didn't match what I saw in my head. I finally thought I looked like a bodybuilder. I had 18" biceps, a pretty big chest, and rather large legs.….I thought I had "arrived." When I would casually talk to people on the street about working out, they would ask me if I did. I would just scratch my head in disbelief. It just made no sense to me that I could bench press a bulldozer but it wasn't obvious to people that I killed myself in the gym. I realized, after this happened to me several times, I needed to change. With this, the quest for reducing my body fat began.

The next fifteen years can be described as an absolute failure. I continued to hit the gym with a new focus on dieting and getting lean. I tried every diet I could get my hands on and even resorted to eating foods that I found utterly disgusting, such as tuna straight from a can. It made me gag but I choked it down in the name of getting lean. I tried no carb, low carb, and low fat, just to name a few, and always managed to lose 15 to 20 pounds before the inevitable would happen. I would grow tired of the deprivation. I missed my pizza and donuts and all the other fun foods I enjoyed. I would cave in once, then twice, and then it was over. Through these vicious cycles, my weight would swing from its height of 255 lbs to a low of 215, but I never managed to stay at my low weight for long. From my low weight, it usually took me a couple years to find my way to the 250s, and then I would get serious and start the cycle all over again.

Enter Russ Branjord and the Spike Diet. I ran across Russ online and fell in love with his attitude toward food and the success he had found, going from fat to lean. I identified with his food struggles he had dealt with his entire life, and wanted to give his program a shot. At the time, I was on another weight loss cycle and weighed around 240 lbs, down from a high of 253 lbs this time around. I didn't know it at the time, but finding Russ was a huge turning point in my life.

I remember planning out my first Spike Day. The menu was full with Chinese food, pizza, donuts, french fries, and candy. All the junk food I was never allowed to eat while dieting was going to be eaten in one day—now this was exciting. To be honest, I overdid it for a while, easily hitting six or seven thousand calories on spike day, but I continued to lose weight. People were amazed at my progress, especially when they witnessed one of my spike days. As the weeks went by, I continued to lose weight weekly. I no longer felt like I was dieting or felt deprived, and I always had my spike day to look forward to every week.

Currently I weigh 203 lbs, which is a weight I haven't seen since I was 17 in high school. I now have people on the street asking me where I work out and if I compete in bodybuilding. My success with my dieting has sparked an interest in me to research dieting and fat loss, and why the Spike Lifestyle works, physiologically. I have even started helping and coaching others on their weight loss journeys and find it very rewarding after struggling with it for so many years.

I continue to lose weight and get stronger in the gym. My bench press is up to 350 lbs, which is an all time high for me, and I achieved this while losing fat. Following the spike diet and its principles, I will soon hit my goal weight of 190 lbs and will finally be, after all these years, big and lean. I am finally in control and I owe it all to Russell Branjord and the Spike Lifestyle.

—Jason F. lost 50 lbs and while building muscle from spiking

112 Pounds Gone and Still Going!

I was obese most of my adult life. Two years ago I took care of my mom as she was dying of cancer. I lived in a fog for a year after that. Then last year I snapped out of it and told myself that I was digging my own grave. I wanted to see my children grow up. I wanted to be healthy and strong and age healthy and strong. On January 11, 2011 I joined myfitnesspal.com and I was weighing an all-time high of 277 pounds and had a BMI of 43.1.

I started following the mainstream, cutting calories sharply and exercising. Yes, the weight was falling off. I had *the bigger you are, the faster you fall* thing going on. But then, I got to a point where I couldn't lose weight. I was doing everything to bust through the plateaus and just remained ever so frustrated. Then I discovered *spiking*. Not only could I have a day to eat food I enjoyed, but it broke my plateaus and kept the scale moving. I no longer live in food-bondage. I'm free to eat the foods I enjoy and lose weight. It's a win-win situation. So exactly one year later, I am 112 pounds lighter. I've gone from squeezing into a size 24 to fitting easily into a size 10. I've got 10 to 15 more pounds to go until I reach my goal, and with spiking I'm going to get there.

P.S. I no longer need my blood pressure meds anymore. I'm FREE

—Cindy lost 112 lbs

Spiker for Life!

I'd been obese ever since I could remember. But when I got to the age of 18, I weighed 282 pounds and I realized I needed to change. That's when my relationship with dieting started. I managed to lose a few pounds, but I never really felt as though I could stay on one of these diets for life. Then I came across the concept of spiking. Eating at a lower calorie goal 6 days a week and high-calorie 1 day a week was a wonderful idea; it means I'm still able to eat all the foods I love whilst still losing weight. Sometimes when I'm eating on my spike day, I think to myself "I'm never going to lose weight eating like this!" But alas, week after week I have continued to drop the pounds. I find a spike day naturally fits into my life as there's usually always 1 day a week when I'm naturally hungrier, and my spike day means I can eat more on that day and still lose weight. Also, after a spike day, I usually can't wait to get back to the healthy eating for the next 6 days! I now weigh 168 pounds and have 18 pounds until I get to my goal weight, I have no doubt spiking will get me there. I'm a spiker for life!

—Lindsey Russell lost 114 lbs spiking!

Spiking is a Lifestyle

I have been overweight for a good portion of my adult life. I've been through a number of different diets. I have done low carb, low fat, low calorie, more exercise, more cardio, more strength, cardio and strength—you name it, I've probably tried it. Every diet I've done in the past ended up with me losing all control due to prolonged strict adherence and having a total breakdown in willpower, leading to a binge of epic proportions that I never recovered from.

I had been using a calorie counting website to track my daily intakes and things were going well so far. However, I was always in fear of falling into my previous pattern of a diet ending in a total caloric blowout that I never recover from. Six months ago, I came across Russell's profile on a calorie counting website's forum. His profile talked about the Spike Diet and how it helped him lose over 100 lbs.

To be honest, I was skeptical at first. After some research and realizing that one of my friends was already using this strategy, I decided to purchase the Kindle version of the Spike Diet book. I was so excited, I read all but the recipes in one sitting and put the strategies to practice that week, and even talked my wife into using them, as well.

I have continued to lose 1.5 to 2.5 pounds weekly since I've started the Spike Lifestyle. Spiking has allowed me to take control of my diet, my health, and my life. I know that once a week I can eat anything I want, so it's that much easier to follow my nutrition plan for the rest of the week. Spike Life isn't a diet! It's a plan for a healthy lifestyle.

—Bruce Delaney lost 56 lbs
Hanover, PA

SPIKE DAY!!!

I clocked in at an all-time high of 382 pounds. I started working out and eating healthy. It was pretty miserable and the weight loss kept slowing down and down and down. I got to around 320 and I had seen the Spike84 talked about on a website I was using for weight loss. So I sent Russell, the author, a private message and then after talking to him, I decided to give Spike84 a try. I am glad I did! During my first week on Spike84, I melted off 5 pounds of weight. When following Spike84, the weight has continued to come off. Since starting Spike84 at 320 pounds, I am now less than 277 pounds for the first time in a very long time! Before   After

The key to this program is that you don't have to suffer or give up food, which is the key for someone like me who is a "foodie." If you exercise just a small amount and follow this eating program (I don't call it a diet, as it's far from what we consider diets) you will lose weight! I love the reactions people who haven't seen me for awhile are having. I've had several people ask me if I had gotten gastric bypass!

All natural—if I can do this, you can do this!

—JR lost nearly 50 lbs with 3 months of spiking

Spike Life Makes Losing Weight Fun

I've struggled with weight my entire life. I can blame it on being overfed when I was young, my genetics, dieting totally destroying my metabolism, or whatever it was, I knew I needed help. I've tried so many different diets, you name it, I've done it, and nothing has worked for me. I remember someone that had observed my battle with weight say, "Maybe you're just supposed to stay this weight forever." I couldn't believe it; it made me more determined than ever to keep trying. One day my friend suggested joining a website to start tracking the calories I was eating. Again, this didn't work for me. Thankfully, though, there I met someone (a life changer), that introduced the Spike Life way of eating to me. Through his counsel, instruction, and knowledge, I followed. I figured I really had exhausted every other way to losing weight that it was worth a shot. The thought of eating whatever I wanted one day a week seemed like it was too good to be true. So I went ahead with it. It took my mind convincing more than anything, and it seemed crazy to eat that much and still be able to lose weight. There I had officially started Spike Life, and had my first Spike Day. I laughed; jumping on the scales and seeing it go up 8 lbs the next day, to then see it drop a few days later. BOOM! There I saw my first 2.2 lbs loss in the longest time I can remember. I cried. I knew this was going to work for me. At a 50 lb loss later, I am continuing this way of life forever. Through this I've learned more than I would have expected, about health and nutrition and what MY body needs and wants. I've learned what it's sensitive toward, and what it soaks up. There's nothing more awesome than knowing you have one heck of a feast, eating WHATEVER you want! (It's only ever six days away!) It almost sounds too good to be true, but it's the only thing that has worked for me. Makes losing weight fun, if you can believe it.

—Katy M. lost 50 lbs
Hong Kong, China

I am Able to Satisfy my Cravings

I guess I am your typical married, mid-30s father of a 19-month-old. I have always been a fairly active person. Having played 4 years of rugby in college, and still have all my faculties! Life threw me and my family a few curveballs in the past few years. Suffice it to say that I was forced to reevaluate my life and where it was heading.

The most important things in my life are my wife and my child. One day I woke up with achy back, sore knees, and no energy for the coming day. I lay in bed and realized I didn't want to be like this for the rest of my life. I had put on close to 50 pounds in one year, through the usage of a new medication and a total lack of diet control. I made a resolution to myself that I needed to be around for my son and wife. I didn't want to leave this Earth too early because I didn't take care of myself. I lost my father when I was 22 and mother when I was 34. I didn't want my son to grow up and lose me or my wife to grow old alone. I knew that something had to be done about my weight and diet.

Thankfully, I came across Russ Branjord and the Spike Lifestyle. I first read about Russ as a personal trainer through Anytime Fitness. In his bio, it said he had lost over 100 lbs in a year through his diet and exercise program. Truthfully, I didn't believe it would happen to me, but I knew he would at least understand where I was coming from with my weight. I started working out with Russ and he told me about his first book, *Spike Diet*, and how it could help me. I was a bit skeptical at first, but was quickly converted to a believer.

Spike Life is something that will work. It will work for the rest of your life; it's not a fad. I have done Atkins and similar diets, and while they work for about a month, they were just not sustainable for me. The Spike Diet is something that changes your dieting habits for your lifetime. Like any other guy, I like pizza and beer. Previously, I had been told to cut those out entirely and say goodbye to my beloved cheese steaks and iced tea. I still watch what I eat during the week, keeping my caloric intake at my targeted goal while maintaining a healthy balanced diet of fruits, veggies, and lean meats. However, when my Spike Day comes (which is Saturday for me) I enjoy all my old favorites. I am able to satisfy my cravings and urges once a week. It's funny, because toward the end of the week, my cravings start to build right about the time I can satisfy them, but during the early part of the week, I tend to crave veggies and fruit. This is a diet plan that guys can use and make part of their life.

Combine the diet with the Spike Life exercise plan and you have an incredible match. Like most guys, I HATE cardio. I don't understand how people can get on a treadmill and run like hamsters in a cage for hours. I am used to running with a definable end point, namely hitting someone. However, you don't see many tackling dummies in gyms. I like how Russ has tailored my exercise program to increase my muscle mass to burn more fat through exercises I enjoy. Russ has done the research and lays out to you, in an understandable fashion, how the science works.

—Andy S.

Army Strong

After seeing the incredible results National Guard Pro Fisherman Mark Courts accomplished, I decided to try the Spike Lifestyle for myself. In less than 3 months I lost over 50 lbs and more than 6 inches from my waist. For the first time in my 17-year career in the National Guard I have been able to maintain myself within the Army's Weight Standards. It was easy. By sticking to the Spike Life meal plan and getting my 10,000 steps a day in, while walking 18 holes at my favorite golf course, I have been able to maintain the weight loss for over 6 months. Spike Life has been a life changing experience for me.

Thank you, Russ, for sharing your awesome plan!

—Troy E. lost 50 lbs and 6 inches off his waist

Story of a girl who took back control and let go of excuses

This girl is 26 years old. She has a husband who has battled cancer (he actually started chemo 2 days after their wedding) and an 8-year-old son who struggles with ADD and some sensory processing issues. Both are a bit on the chunky side. She's been through quite a lot in her young life, dealing with everything from severe abuse to serious mental health issues that have, on more than one occasion, resulted in hospitalization. She was diagnosed with clinical depression at age 11 and, later on, was diagnosed as bipolar.

Life hasn't been easy for this girl, and it's taken its toll. She's been obese for about 6 years now. She's tired all of the time. Her feet are always swollen and her joints ache. She's depressed.

She has almost 56% body fat and wears 24W pants, XXL shirts, and 20W dresses.

This girl feels closer to 62 than 26.

So the girl goes to the doctor to see about her depression meds and the doctor recommends, in addition to a different medication, adding some exercise to her day to help release some endorphins.

This girl hates exercise—she is, after all, quite heavy and her knees and feet and ankles and basically her entire body hurt when she tries to be active.

But then she thinks: "If I have to be active to be healthier emotionally, why not go all out and get healthy physically, too?"

So she does.

She dumps the junk from her house. She stocks up on fresh fruits and veggies, lean proteins, healthy fats, whole grains, and other nutritious foods. She stops chugging lemonade and starts drinking water instead.

And she gets her body moving.

At first, it's tough. She's in such terrible shape that all she can manage is a walk around her neighborhood and, quite honestly, the junk food was a bit of an addiction. It's hard to give up, but when she's tempted, she reminds herself of this.

So she makes the right choices, whether she feels like it or not.

Gradually, things get easier. She starts learning (and, surprisingly, enjoying) new recipes and finds ways to cook old favorites to make them healthier. She increases her endurance and speed when walking. She adds some new exercises.

And her body starts to change.

At first, it's not that noticeable. The girl is quite tall, you see, which means it takes a bit more for weight gain or loss to show. Still, things do start changing.

Her feet stop swelling. Her double chin starts shrinking. She notices that it's more comfortable to fit into the auditorium seats at church. There's a bit more room between her belly and the steering wheel. It's easier to tie her shoes.

The girl is consistent and more changes happen. Collarbones appear. She gets out of the Plus Sized section at the store. She doesn't struggle as much to keep up during fitness classes. She has more energy.

She keeps going, keeps focusing on getting healthy, getting fit, and setting a good example for her family.

A year later, the girl I introduced you to at the beginning of this story is gone. A new girl has replaced her. This is the girl I want to tell you about now:

This girl is 27 years old. Like the girl mentioned earlier, she has a husband who, thank God, is still cancer-free, and a now-9-year-old son who still struggles with ADD and some other issues. The hubby and son are still a bit chubby, but they are a lot more active now.

This girl, like the one in the beginning of the story, has gone through abuse and mental health challenges and all sorts of other things that she decided she wouldn't let hurt her anymore.

She decided that she was going to take control and get healthy. She doesn't use her past as an excuse for bad choices and doesn't let her obstacles daunt her—she overcomes them, one step at a time.

This girl loves exercise. She loves eating healthy foods and making healthy meals for family and friends. She is fit and healthy and (usually) has tons of energy. She's still bipolar, but her symptoms are about a million times better than they've ever been before.

She has 23% body fat, wears size 8 pants, Small (and even occasionally Extra Small) shirts.

So who is that girl, anyway? It's me!

I am so glad I made the decision to change the way I live my life, to replace my unhealthy habits, laziness and gluttony, with regular exercise and proper nutrition and healthy portions. I passed my weight loss goal of 100 pounds about a month and a half ago and, as of today I have shed 125 pounds and around 90 inches from all over my body. In turn, I have also gained some things: good health, confidence, and the knowledge that I am setting a positive example for my family and friends.

—Cory A. lost 126 lbs and 90 inches by changing her lifestyle

Breaking the Diet Plateau

I started the Spike Lifestyle after a friend told me about your book, and I'd tried multiple ways to break a 6-MONTH plateau!

Nothing worked and I had come too far to quit (only 8 lbs shy of my goal weight).

We started doing Spike together December 30, my birthday, and I cannot be more thrilled!

I have finally broken this dreadful plateau by using your approach!

Thank you so much.

—Krystal

SPIKE DIET CUSTOMER REVIEWS

I'm so Glad I Found This!

I found after 6 months of steady weight loss, and then several months of doing the same things but **not** losing any more weight, that Spiking was right for me!

Other than very general guidelines, this is not the kind of "diet" that lays out weird specific foods for you or puts an entire food group on the naughty list (although there are several recipes to get the ideas flowing). You can make your plan of whatever healthy foods you choose. That part is just common sense and good nutrition.

The magic is in the math: you do a little bit to figure out where your calories should be for the various days of the week. You have three days at a lower rate, three days at a medium rate, and one ridiculously awesome day—your Spike Day—at a really high calorie limit. HIGH, really-really high! It's all laid out for you and is quite simple once you plug in your own info.

The idea is that overall, your week is a deficit so you lose weight, while the Spike Day tells your body that there's no need to panic and lower your metabolism. I'm pretty sure that's what happened to me—I was at a lowered calorie limit for so long that it adjusted my metabolism to match. Hell, no—not standing for that!

Although it wasn't really my issue, there's another cool aspect of this plan—people who have a hard time with feeling deprived on lower calories have that reset switch on Spike Day. Anyone can do anything for six days at a time, right?! If you're really craving something that's considered not weight-loss friendly, you never have more than six days until you can indulge. It's crazy.

Since I got the book and put it into action, I've begun losing weight again at a healthy clip and I'm feeling good about it. And it's really funny to see something that would normally be considered way too far outside weight-loss boundaries (my first Spike Day purchase was a fried pie, like those gross Hostess things) and be able to buy it and set it aside for later. You feel weird at first, but trust me—you get over it. When I explain this plan to someone, they almost always say, "How fun!" and that's exactly it: it IS fun!

This totally put me back on track to my goals—thanks, Russell!

It Works!

I have to agree with all of the 5-Star reviews! *Spike Diet* is a quick read and very informative. It was really easy and fun to read, also. I keep reading it over and over. I have lost 10.5 lbs and 4 inches off my waist in just under 2 weeks of spiking. I have tried many diets over the years and the Spike Lifestyle is the only one that works for me. I have recommended this to all my friends and family. I had been "dieting" for over a year prior, with slow process, and I hit the dreaded plateau. Spiking has helped me breakthrough and start losing again. A++++

It Really Does Work!

I have lost 18 lbs so far in 6 weeks with no sign of slowing down! The book is great, a quick easy read. And I love that I never feel deprived because I can eat it on my spike day. I have so much more energy now!

What a Concept!

I read *Spike Diet* at just the right time. Stuck at the inevitable dieters' plateau, I found this book, and I personally have dropped 5.6 lbs in the first two weeks on it. The idea makes perfect sense, considering metabolism and calories in vs. calories out. It is explained matter-of-factly in a short, easy to understand read. The author gets right to the point, explaining how the Spike Diet works, and how he used it to lose 100 lbs. This book is useful to anyone wanting to lose weight, and who knows the dreaded dieters' plateau.

Have your Cake and Eat it Too!

Enter the *Spike Diet*. This book takes out all the BS filler most diet books are stuffed with and gives you what you need to know. You can actually sit down, start reading, and get everything you need to know in one session. I've been interested in diet/fitness for years, and reading this book just flipped the "AHA!" switch in my head. I had previously implemented several of the strategies in the book during my journey to better health, but had never thought about how much synergy these ideas had until I started reading.

I wanted to wait at least 2 weeks of following the program exactly to give a review. In that time I've gone from a starting weight of 202 to 196. Six pounds may not seem like a lot to some people, but most sources recommend losing 1-2 pounds a week. If you're overweight, just imagine where you'd be if you lost one pound every week for a year. It's especially impressive to me since I was stuck on a serious plateau, and I lost weight while eating foods that are usually considered "forbidden" for dieters. I like that this diet has a transition to maintenance, so that you keep your weight off. I also like that it doesn't go completely crazy.

Even though you're eating a lot of calories on the Spike Day, there is still a calorie goal. No diet that lets you eat ten pizzas a day will work, but because the "limit" is so high, you'll have a hard time hitting it. I had trouble getting in all my calories on the Spike Day because I was stuffed. I didn't have to worry about temptation because I knew I could have basically whatever I wanted on that day. If I saw something "bad" I just got it, saved it until Spike Day, and ate it with zero guilt. As an example, on my first Spike Day I had two cake doughnuts, one apple fritter, a bottle of chocolate milk, and two sausage McGriddles for breakfast. A grand total of 2,000 just for my FIRST meal of the day, and I still lost weight. To be honest, I love junk food and probably always will, but you don't have to eat junk on your Spike Day. You can still eat completely healthy if you want as long as you get the extra calories in.

Pure Genius!

Spike Diet puts it all together. I now know why I stopped losing weight. I am now losing weight again and it's never been easier. If you are on a diet plateau, this is the book for you. Even if you're happy with your current diet, this is still the book for you!

It will forever change your views on food and dieting. Spike Day is the greatest day ever for a dieter, and with the awesome recipes in the book, it is easy to stay on track the other 6 days.

Spiking Works!

I was skeptical, but my friend urged me to try the Spike Diet, claiming it was the magic behind her weight loss. I didn't understand how eating cookies and pizza would help me lose weight, but I took her word on it, mostly because I could see her success.

The book was very quick and easy to read, and while some of the science went over my head, I was still able to get a firm grasp on metabolism and "starvation mode." It was starvation mode and depriving myself that was behind my past failed attempts at losing weight. My first Spike Day, I was kind of afraid to give in, but once I started with waffles and a donut I was off to the races. I lost 3-4 pounds each and every week, and all of a sudden the Spike Diet started making sense. My energy levels were up, and I was feeling great, which has never happened before while I was on a diet. It was also great having Spike Days during the Holiday season, so I could eat whatever I wanted on Thanksgiving, and I will be doing the same on Christmas. I'm now only 15 pounds from my goal weight, and it has been a rather easy ride to get where I am now, so I am certain I will hit my goal weight soon after New Year's, when most people are just starting their weight-loss resolutions. I highly recommend this book!

"Starvation Mode" is a thing in the past!

I've lost 70 lbs already!

The method is truly amazing and it's backed by real science of how our body's metabolism works. I've tried everything in the past, and like everyone, I am a skeptic. When I saw the book at my gym, and read an article in our paper about the author, I took a chance on the Spike Diet, and I am so happy I did—it has changed my life.

There is nothing really restricted on the diet; it's just based off of simple calorie intake versus our calories burned, so I could eat fruit or bread every day. I just had a calorie goal to reach; for me it was around 1,800 calories so I never felt hungry or deprived.

Then once a week I was able to eat whatever I wanted, without guilt. I was able to fully enjoy what I was eating because I knew that my Spike Day was about to turn me into a "fat-burning machine" for the following week.

Overall, I have lost 70 pounds, in about 7 months, and I am only 10 pounds away from my goal weight and my size 6 dress!

It really helped knowing that the author has lost over 100 pounds and the book speaks of his struggles and experience. It really made me feel like I could do it, and I did!

Eat what I want AND lose weight?! Yes please!

I was obviously skeptical when I started my new Spike Lifestyle, but this book explains the science very simply. It is right to the point, and it makes a LOT of sense! Stick to your calorie goals for 6 days, get to eat whatever on that 7th day, see the pounds drop off! The best part? There is no sprinkling mystery chemicals on your food, no prepackaged diet foods (unless you dig that sort of thing), no restricting carbs, or meat, or dairy, or solids, no specific recipes you have to follow, no nonsense! This "diet" isn't a fad diet. This is a lifestyle change—you can do this for the rest of your life, while never having to feel deprived or isolated. If you are tired of dieting, and tired of feeling deprived, and tired of being overweight, buy this book and try it. You won't be sorry.

Diet, exercise, and PIZZA in the same sentence!?

I am probably your typical dieter. . . I step on the scale, see a nasty number, VOW to change, diet perfectly for 2-3 weeks, then fall miserably back into my old routines—inevitably regaining any weight I lost and a few extra pounds to boot! I joined an online weight loss group and started to head in the right direction again. . . then felt myself slipping again. . . AARGH! I happened to come across a "before and after" picture of someone and decided to send them a message. They told me about spiking and I ordered the book the same night! Took all of half an hour to read it (I hate books that take FOREVER to get to the actual diet). I have been spiking ever since, dropping anywhere from 2-5 pounds a week. Russell has been GREAT every step of the way! I followed the plan very loosely at first, but lately I have been adding in the exercising and the plan works either way! So if you dread the idea of a strict plan to follow at all times, this is the plan for you! It's a way of life now for me. I can diet all week long, knowing that my Spike Day is coming up soon. I actually find myself looking forward to eating healthy the day after. (I NEVER thought I'd be the one to spit those words out!) Still skeptical? Buy the book, try it for a week or two, and let the results convince you! Sometimes seeing is believing—and I am a TRUE believer!

Just Started this "Lifestyle"

I have been on the weight loss journey for a LONG time. I lose and gain a touch back, lose and gain a touch back. I was never really able to find something that fit my life. I am VERY structured during the week and don't find it difficult. Eating is bang on, workouts are great, but Saturday is my issue. Nothing is routine. No gym, no regular meals, and kids at home. I have been searching for a plan I could live with realistically and finally came across Russell's book and I have begun following this lifestyle. That is the key: it is a LIFESTYLE. It FITS my lifestyle! I don't have to make it fit. 6 days a week I am structured and the 7th day...well, you got to see it to believe it. You actually HAVE to enjoy yourself to make the plan work—no more horribly guilty feelings for indulging a bit. It is REQUIRED!!

So far, I LOVE it and Russ is a great, helpful guy! He understands where we are coming from, weight-wise and loving food. Lots of "yummy, why should I deprive myself" food! I highly recommend this program to everyone who enjoys food like I do, has the desire to follow calories during the week, and spends family and friend time over the weekend—make it SPIKE time! Highly recommend!

Skeptic to Believer

Before I started reading *Spike*, I was like most people, who think, "Yeah, right, there is no way you can lose weight and splurge, that's a recipe for disaster." After taking the time to read through everything Russell had to say, I realized that it is completely possible. I read the book twice, did some research online, talked to friends who were doing it, and was convinced this was my best choice. I haven't regretted my decision at all.

Knowing that I can eat healthy all week and have one "splurge" day is amazing for willpower and cravings. Once those urges are gone, I can't wait to get back to my healthy eating. This has helped break my weight loss plateau as well as give me a new perspective on healthy living in general.

Russell does a great job explaining how Spike works and why it's beneficial to anyone. There is no set "you have to eat this, this, and this." It's very flexible; the calculations are easy to understand and make sense. I've suggested it to many friends having trouble with living a healthy lifestyle and will continue to. **Changed my life and how I look at food...Forever**

This book changed my life. It's straightforward and tells you EXACTLY what you need to do to lose weight. Another thing you can do is go online to Facebook and like "The Spike Diet" page and ask him any questions you want. HE WILL ANSWER YOU. Buy this because the guy who wrote it isn't just selling his product, he believes in it, and actually DOES IT. I've done this for 3 months now and lost 35 lbs. Thanks, Russ!

Easiest and most doable diet I have been on

I tried for a year working out like crazy, trying to lose the last 10 pounds, but what I was doing did not work. The Spike Diet did work for me and I think after the first week of getting the hang of it, it is the easiest diet I have been on. I plan for it to be the way I eat and live for the rest of my life. My grocery cost has not gone up; I just choose different items and actually buy a little less. The recipes are super delicious and keep me from getting too hungry. I have had a couple of slip-ups and it has not affected me, as I get back on it the next day. I am not saying this is smooth sailing—there are tough moments, but knowing I have a Spike day coming up helps me choose the right foods during the week.

I have lost a size and a half in two months and have maintained it for eight months. I now fit into clothes that have not fit me since my wedding. I am also close to a size I have not worn since I do not even remember, maybe eighth grade? I hope to be fully in that size by the end of August.

I am a busy mom, actress and singer so I do not have much time for workouts, but I can fit ten minutes a day in and a more intense workout once a week. What a great diet and way to live! Thanks, Russ!

APPENDIX

SPIKE LIFE QUICK-START GUIDE

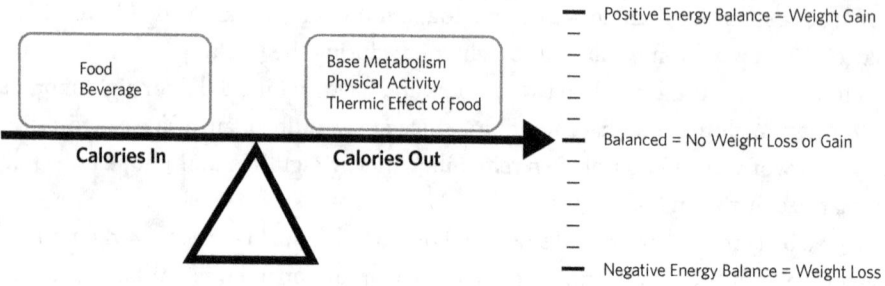

Losing Weight is: Calories In Versus Calories Out

Spike Life creates a weekly caloric deficit while keeping hormones balanced and metabolism strong.

SPIKE LIFE QUICK-START STEPS
1. Find your calorie range
2. Plan your meals
3. Record your meals in a food journal
4. Exercise at least one hour a week
5. Be active daily
6. Enjoy your Spike Day

FIRST—FIND YOUR DAILY CALORIE RANGE

We need to create a caloric deficit to force our body to burn fat.

SPIKE LIFE CALORIE TARGETS

MEN			WOMEN		
Body Weight	Calorie Range	Spike day Calories	Body Weight	Calorie Range	Spike day Calories
170lbs	1400-1900	3800	20lbs	1200-1300	2600
180lbs	1440-1950	3900	130lbs	1200-1350	2700
190lbs	1500-2000	4000	140lbs	1200-1400	2800
200lbs	1550-2050	4100	150lbs	1200-1450	2900
210lbs	1600-2100	4200	160lbs	1200-1500	3000
220lbs	1650-2150	4300	170lbs	1200-1550	3100
230lbs	1700-2200	4400	180lbs	1200-1600	3200
240lbs	1750-2250	4500	190lbs	1200-1650	3300
250lbs	1800-2300	4600	200lbs	1200-1700	3400
260lbs	1850-2350	4700	210lbs	1225-1725	3500
270lbs	1900-2400	4800	220lbs	1250-1750	3500
280lbs	1950-2450	4900	230lbs	1300-1800	3500
290lbs	2000-2500	5000	240lbs	1325-1825	3500
300lbs	2050-2550	5000	250lbs	1350-1850	3500
310lbs	2100-2600	5000	260lbs	1400-1900	3500
320bs	2150-2650	5000	270lbs	1425-1925	3500
330lbs	2200-2700	5000	280lbs	1450-1950	3500
340lbs	2250-2750	5000	290lbs	1500-2000	3500
350+lbs	2300-2800	5000	300+lbs	1550-2050	3500

Six days stay within your calorie range and one day a week enjoy a Spike Day!

SECOND—PLAN YOUR DAILY MENUS
Choose foods that provide nutritional value, satiety, and a metabolic boost.

Spike Life Food Pyramid

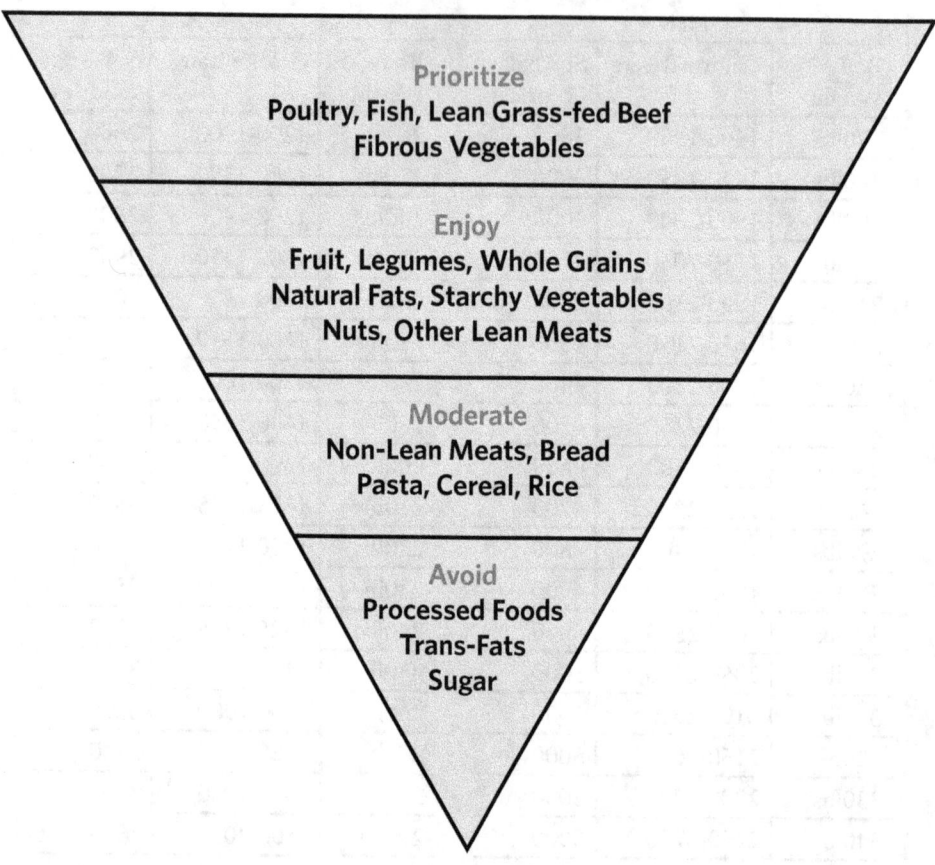

Prioritize
Poultry, Fish, Lean Grass-fed Beef
Fibrous Vegetables

Enjoy
Fruit, Legumes, Whole Grains
Natural Fats, Starchy Vegetables
Nuts, Other Lean Meats

Moderate
Non-Lean Meats, Bread
Pasta, Cereal, Rice

Avoid
Processed Foods
Trans-Fats
Sugar

Prioritize—Every Meal
Moderate—One or Two Meals a Day
Enjoy—Half of Daily Meals
Avoid—Limit to Spike Day

SPIKE LIFE FOOD LIST

FOODS TO EAT:	FOODS TO AVOID:
Grass-fed beef	Processed foods
Fish	Trans-fats
Poultry	Snack cakes
Other lean meat	Cookies
Vegetables	Fast-foods
High fiber foods	Sugar
Beans and legumes	White bread
Nuts	White pasta
Eggs	Vegetable oil
Milk	Hydrogenated oils
Reduced fat cheese	Margarine
Fruits	Butter
Oats	Shortening
Whole grains	High sugar cereals
Bran	High fructose corn syrup
Quinoa	Sugary beverages
Olive oil	Soda
Coconut oil	Juice
Coconut flour	Cream latte's
Organic honey	Ice cream
Agave	Frozen meals
Avocados	
Sweet potatoes	

Eat a balanced diet high in protein and fiber.

34% proteins—33% carbohydrates—33% Dietary Fat

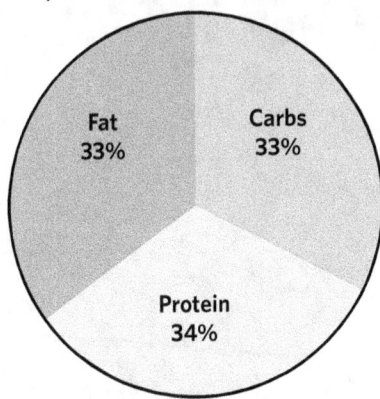

*Another important goal is to get 30-50 grams of fiber daily. Fiber with every meal will help to stabilize blood sugar and control our hunger.

GRAMS PER DAILY CALORIE GOAL

Calories	Fat Grams	Carbs Grams	Protein Grams
1200	44	99	102
1300	48	107	110
1400	51	116	119
1500	55	124	128
1600	59	132	136
1700	62	140	145
1800	66	149	153
1900	70	157	162
2000	73	165	170

Use this chart as a guide for your daily meal plan.

Calories X 34% / 4 = Protein Grams
Calories X 33% / 4 = Carbohydrate Grams
Calories X 33% / 9 = Fat Grams

Use this chart as a guide for your daily meal plan.

Calories X 34% / 4 = Protein Grams
Calories X 33% / 4 = Carbohydrate Grams
Calories X 33% / 9 = Fat Grams

THIRD—RECORD YOUR MEALS IN A FOOD JOURNAL
Dieters who log their meals lose twice as much weight as those who don't.

	MEAL	CALORIES	FAT	CARBS	FIBER	PROTEIN
BREAKFAST						
SNACK						
LUNCH						
SNACK						
DINNER						
SNACK						
TOTAL						

CALORIE DIARY

FOURTH—EXERCISE AT LEAST ONE HOUR A WEEK
All types of exercise burn extra calories.

▸ Find an exercise you enjoy doing
▸ Strength training is the best for fat-burning
▸ HIIT cardio is effective and can be done at home

SPIKE LIFE HOME HIIT WORKOUT

1. WARM-UP: Very Important

EXERCISE	TIME	REST (WALK IN PLACE)
Jumping Jacks	30 seconds	30 seconds
High Knees	30 seconds	30 seconds
Wall Push-Ups	30 seconds	30 seconds

2. REST AN EXTRA MINUTE AND THEN BEGIN

3. SPIKE LIFE HIGH INTENSITY INTERVAL TRAINING: REPEAT 2-3 TIMES

EXERCISE	TIME	REST
Push-Ups	40 seconds	30 seconds
High Knees	40 seconds	30 seconds
Burpees	40 seconds	30 seconds
Jump Squats	40 seconds	30 seconds
Jumping Jacks	40 seconds	30 seconds

The Spike Life Home HIIT workout takes between 10-20 minutes based on the number of repetitions you complete. Depending on your exercise levels you may want to just complete one full round or take a longer rest period between exercises. It's better to start out slow and work your way up. You can find descriptions and videos if these exercises at spikelifebook.com.

FIFTH—BE ACTIVE DAILY

By being more active on a daily basis, we increase our metabolism and burn calories through NEAT (Non-Exercise Activity Thermogenesis).

Daily Goal of 10,000 Steps

Here are some simple ideas to incorporate 10,000 steps into your daily routine.

- ▶ Take a thirty minute walk after dinner.
- ▶ Use the stairs instead of the elevator.
- ▶ Walk the dog.
- ▶ At stores, park in the back end of the parking lot.
- ▶ Walk to the store.
- ▶ Get up to change the channel.
- ▶ Shop at malls or outdoor outlet malls.
- ▶ Plan a neighborhood walking group.
- ▶ Walk over to visit a neighbor.
- ▶ Get outside to walk around the garden or do a little weeding.
- ▶ Play games with your kids.
- ▶ Play active video games, like dance games.
- ▶ Walk on a treadmill while you watch TV.
- ▶ Jump on a mini-trampoline and listen to your favorite music.
- ▶ At work, get up off your chair and walk around during breaks.
- ▶ Make being active a daily priority .

SIXTH—ENJOY YOUR SPIKE DAY
Spike Days raise leptin levels, boosting metabolism and reducing cravings. This allows you to be control over your body instead of food.

Spiking never allows our body adapt to a lower calorie intake
Before our metabolism gets a chance to adapt, we have a Spike Day. It sends an *emphatic* message to our brain that we are not in the middle of a famine. Our body then goes back to burning calories and fat as usual.

Spike Days raise leptin and crush food cravings after we spike
Spike Days increase our leptin levels, making us feel satisfied and destroying the cravings that were beginning to have an effect on us.

Spike Days actually spike metabolism!
The calorie surplus from spiking causes the body to increase our basal metabolic rate (BMR) about 9% above baseline, and it's hypothesized that more is possible.

Spike Days improve your workouts
Spike Days allow us to restore our muscle glycogen, the stored glucose in our muscles used to fuel our workouts. Glycogen is often depleted when we diet, and restoring it will provide excellent results for our workouts following Spike Day.

Spike Days give us a mental break from all things diet related
Who truly loves dieting? I sure don't. Spike Life gives you a break every week from dieting, so you are able to come back fresh and renewed—mentally, hormonally, and physically.

BMI INDEX CHARTS

WEIGHT	140	150	160	170	180	190	200	210	230	230	240	250
BODY MASS INDEX (BMI) CHART												

HEIGHT	WEIGHT	140	150	160	170	180	190	200	210	230	230	240	250
	5'0"	27	29	31	33	35	37	39	41	43	45	47	49
	5'3"	25	27	28	30	32	34	36	37	39	41	43	44
	5'6"	23	24	26	28	29	31	32	34	36	37	39	40
	5'9"	21	22	24	25	27	28	30	31	33	34	36	37
	6'0"	19	20	22	23	25	26	27	29	30	31	33	34
	6'3"	18	19	20	21	23	24	25	26	28	29	30	31

BMI RANGES

BMI	Status
Below 18.5	Underweight
18.5—24.9	Normal
25.0—29.9	Overweight
30.0—40.0	Obese
40.0—54.0+	Extremely Obese

BMR CHART

MEN WEIGHT	BMR		WOMEN WEIGHT	BMR
170lbs	1900		120lbs	1300
180lbs	1950		130lbs	1350
190lbs	2000		140lbs	1400
200lbs	2050		150lbs	1450
210lbs	2100		160lbs	1500
220lbs	2150		170lbs	1550
230lbs	2200		180lbs	1600
240lbs	2250		190lbs	1650
250lbs	2300		200lbs	1700
260lbs	2350		210lbs	1725
270lbs	2400		220lbs	1750
280lbs	2450		230lbs	1800
290lbs	2500		240lbs	1825
300lbs	2550		250lbs	1850
310lbs	2600		260lbs	1900
320bs	2650		270lbs	1925
330lbs	2700		280lbs	1950
340lbs	2750		290lbs	2000
350+lbs	2800		300+lbs	2050

TOTAL DAILY ENERGY EXPENDITURE
Total Daily Energy Expenditure (TDEE) = (BMR) X (Activity Multiplier)

Activity Multipliers
Sedentary = BMR x 1.2 (little or no exercise or activity)
Lightly Active = BMR x 1.375 (exercise and activity 1-3 days/week)
Moderately Active = BMR x 1.55 (exercise and activity 3-5 days/week)
Very Active = BMR x 1.725 (exercise and activity 6-7 days/week)
Extremely Active = BMR x 1.9 (daily exercise or physical job)

PREDICT YOUR WEEKLY FAT LOSS WORKSHEET
Use the charts in this chapter and the examples above

PREDICT YOUR WEEKLY FAT LOSS WORKSHEET

Use the charts in this chapter and the examples above

TOTAL CALORIES EXPENDED = TDEE (BMR X ACTIVITY MULTIPLIER)

BMR	
X (Activity Multiplier)	
TDEE	
Calories Burned Daily	
Calories Burned Weekly	

TOTAL CALORIES CONSUMED:

Calorie Range (from chart)	*calories*
Three "Low Days"	X 3(days) =
Three "High Days"	X 3(days) =
Spike Day	calories

TOTAL "CALORIES IN" VS. "CALORIES OUT" FOR THE WEEK:

Total "Calories In"	calories consumed weekly
Total "Calories Out"	calories burned weekly
Net Weekly Calorie Deficit	calories

TOTAL PROJECTED FAT LOSS:

_____ /3500= _____ lbs fat loss per week/ _____ lbs year

(One Pound of Fat equals 3,500 Calories)

If you're not satisfied with your predicted weight loss, you can have more days in the lower range of your calorie goals and exercise more often. Remember, Spike Life is about living a manageable healthy lifestyle where you can lose weight and maintain your weight loss. This is not a "crash diet" designed to lose a bunch of weight up front and put you in a position where it's impossible to maintain it. We are stopping the insanity and losing weight in a fun and healthy way.

FOOD FULLNESS GRADES

FOODS GRADED ON FULLNESS PER CALORIE

A+
Bean sprouts
Watermelon
Grapefruit
Carrots
Broccoli

A
Oranges
Fish, broiled
Grilled chicken
Apples
Sirloin steak

B+
Popcorn
Baked potato
Greek yogurt
Banana
High fiber Cereal

B
Quinoa
Brown rice
Low fat yogurt
Fiber bars
Rolled oats

C+
Spaghetti
Macaroni & Cheese
Cereal & Milk

C
Pizza
White Rice
Peanuts

D+
Ice cream
White bread
Raisins

D
Candy Bar
Honey

F
Sugar
Potato chips
Snack cakes
Butter
Soda
Juice
Oils

SPIKE LIFE GROCERY SHOPPING LIST

- Low-Carb Tortillas
- Low-Carb Flax, Oat, and Wheat Pitas
- Low-Carb Flat Breads
- Low-Fat Liquid Egg Substitutes
- Low-Fat or 2% Cheese Slices, Shredded, & Sticks
- Extra Lean Ground Turkey
- Lean Grass-Fed Beef, Fresh & Frozen
- Light Hamburger Buns
- Light Bread (40-45 calories per slice with added fiber)
- Natural & Lean Deli Meat
- Beef Jerky
- Fiber Snack Bars
- Fresh Fruit and Vegetables (from local farmer markets)
- Frozen Organic Fruit
- Frozen Veggies (single servings)
- Light Sour Cream
- Coconut Oil
- Coconut Milk Ice Cream
- Organic Ketchup (no high fructose corn syrup)
- Canadian Bacon
- Natural Peanut Butter
- Low-Carb Protein Shakes
- Pre-Grilled Chicken
- Natural and Reduced-Carb Breaded Chicken Breasts
- Olive Oil Reduced-Fat Mayo

LOWER CALORIE SNACKS IDEAS

- ▸ Beef & Turkey Jerky
- ▸ Low-Fat Cheese Sticks (2%)
- ▸ Protein Shakes: use 4oz of milk and 4oz of low-fat liquid egg replacement, blend with ice in a blender. Add chocolate—the result is delicious like a chocolate malt.
- ▸ Hard-Boiled and Deviled Eggs
- ▸ Pickles
- ▸ Sugar-Free Pudding
- ▸ Sugar-Free Frozen Fudge Bars
- ▸ Green Veggies
- ▸ Deli Meat
- ▸ Lean Meats: turkey, chicken, venison, lean beef, and bison
- ▸ Turkey Pepperoni with reduced-fat parmesan cheese sprinkled on top
- ▸ Deli Meat with reduced-fat cream cheese, wrapped in a low-carb tortilla
- ▸ Peanut Butter and Celery
- ▸ Nuts
- ▸ Soy Beans
- ▸ Low-Carb Protein Bars
- ▸ Low-Carb Shakes, ready-to-drink·
- ▸ Breakfast Pizza, using low-carb flatbreads
- ▸ Breakfast Burritos, using low-carb tortillas

CALORIE DIARY

MEAL	CALORIES	FAT	CARBS	FIBER	PROTEIN
BREAKFAST					
SNACK					
LUNCH					
SNACK					
DINNER					
SNACK					
TOTAL					

FAILURE & BURN WORKOUT (BLANK)

Muscle Group: _____ : 20-30 Minutes

Going to "failure" is key for progression and "burning out" is important for recovery

ORDER	EXERCISE	MUSCLES TRAINED	SET 1	SET 2	SET 3
ONE-SET "FAILURE" EXERCISES (REST 60 SECONDS BETWEEN EXERCISES)					
1			Warm-up	Warm-up	*
2			Warm-up	Warm-up	*
3			SKIP	Warm-up	*
4			SKIP	Warm-up	*
SPIKE "BURN" GAUNTLET (NO REST - TO FAILURE WITH LIGHTER RESISTANCE)					
5			12-20 reps	12-20 reps	12-20 reps
6			12-20 reps	12-20 reps	12-20 reps
7			12-20 reps	12-20 reps	12-20 reps
8			12-20 reps	12-20 reps	12-20 reps

* 6-9 rep range for advanced lifters and 10-15 for beginners (See trainer tips below)

SPIKE LIFE TIPS

Work Out at Home & Gym

I have both a gym membership and home exercise equipment so I have the option to do both, depending on my free time and the workout. I find most of my home exercise equipment cheap at garage sales, local online sales listings sites, and online auction sites. After the New Year, I typically find a flood of listings for hardly used exercise equipment for less than half the cost of new.

Use a Spotter

You should always have a trained spotter helping you when you exercise to failure with free weights.

Building a Six-Pack

Rectus Abdominus is actually one large muscle, but different movements put the focus on either the lower or upper part of the abdominal muscle. I perform different exercises to accentuate development in both my upper and lower abs. Pulling your legs to your body triggers your lower abs and hip flexors. While crunching your upper body down to your core, like a sit-up, triggers your upper abdominal region. Obliques are the muscles on our sides underneath the preverbal "love handles." In order to build a great six-pack, you need to work all aspects of your core, including your lower back, for muscle balance and stability. I train my abdominals the same way I train every other muscle: with resistance to reach the muscle failure point in the 6-12 rep range. In the past I would do thousands of crunches with nothing to show for it, but once I started using resistance so I could only complete about a dozen reps before muscle failure, my six-pack started to appear. Since our body loves to store body fat in our core, no matter how strong your abs are, you won't see a thing until your diet is under control and you burn fat from that area. If you are overweight you should still do core exercises because your six-pack will be there waiting for you when the fat has been melted away.

Maximize Glycogen Loading

To maximize the glycogen loading effect of spiking: reduce your carbohydrate intake three days prior to your Spike Day, and when you spike, eat 60% of your Spike Day calories from carbohydrates. This isn't a necessity for weight loss but it further enhances the exercise benefits of spiking.

Alcohol

You should avoid mixing high calorie foods with alcohol. When we drink alcohol while eating food, our body makes metabolizing alcohol calories the priority to get them out of our system as fast as possible. In the meantime, the foods that we consume have a higher probability of being stored as fat.

Coconut Oil

Coconut oil is mostly saturated fat, but it's a unique type of fat called MCTs or medium-chain-triglycerides. MCTs are sent directly to the liver and converted to energy and cannot be stored as body fat. They can actually stimulate our metabolism and help us lose weight. Coconut oil is the best kind of fat for health and losing weight. Since coconut oil is perfect for high-heat use, I use it to cook, fry, and bake my meals.

Olive Oil

I love mayonnaise on food so I use olive oil mayo instead of regular mayo to get more oleic acid in my diet.

Resistant Starch

A green banana contains 12.5 grams of resistant starch.

High GI Food

Adding protein and fiber to high GI foods slows the digestion and lessens the impact on our blood sugar and insulin.

Cravings

I carry mint gum with me to stop me from giving in to food temptations when my cravings are aroused by the smell or sight of my favorite foods. Chewing mint gum will ruin the flavor of anything and a second of willpower to pop gum in my mouth stops me from grabbing food I really don't want to have.

After-Spike Workouts

Spike Days restore muscle glycogen, so the day after spiking we have enhanced endurance and strength for our workouts.

Avoiding Hunger Between Meals

Drinking water between meals can reduce ghrelin and hunger. For an even better effect add fiber powder to your water.

Protein and Fiber Make Us Feel Full

High protein and fiber foods provide a very high level of satiety. These foods need to become the staples of our diet.

Food Labeled "Low-Fat" Doesn't Mean It's Healthy

I often choose "reduced-fat" options for foods because they generally have less overall calories than the full-fat version. However, some food manufactures replace the fat with sugar or HFCS; these options I avoid and choose the regular full-fat version. This is where reading food labels is very important. If the reduced-fat version has the same number of calories than the original, then it usually has added calories from sugar. Just remember: a food labeled "low-fat" doesn't mean it's healthy.

Dietary Fats Are Essential to Health

Dietary fats are needed to produce key sex hormones that promote healthy weight and anti-aging.

Choose Grass-Fed Beef for High Levels of Omega-3s

The recommended ratio of consumption for Omega-3 fatty acids and Omega-6 fatty acids is 4-to-1. Grass-fed beef has an Omega-3 to Omega-6 ratio of 3:1, while grain-fed beef has a ratio of 20:1.

THESE ARE A FEW OF MY FAVORITE THINGS...

My Favorite Exercise
Bench Press

My Favorite Workout Song
"Bodies" by Drowning Pool

My Favorite Spike Day Food
Cinnamon Persian Donuts with cream cheese frosting

My Favorite Non-Spike Day Food
Turkey Flat Bread Sandwich with center-cut bacon and olive oil mayo, fried with co-conut oil.

My Favorite Choice for Bacon
Center-Cut Bacon—It has less fat than turkey bacon but still tastes like the real thing, and I love bacon!

My Favorite Protein Powder
Trutein in CinnaBun flavor—Amazing nutritional profile and even better taste

My Favorite Ready-To-Drink Protein Shake
EAS Carb Control Chocolate Fudge—17 grams of protein and only 110 calories

My Favorite Day to Spike
Saturday—It's a great way to start the weekend, and I have Sunday to go to the gym for my after-spike workout.

My Favorite Non-Spike Fitness Book
It's the first one I ever bought: *The New Encyclopedia of Modern Bodybuilding* by Arnold Schwarzenegger.

My Favorite Thing to Do with Free Time
Playing hide and seek and wrestling with my three boys.

My Favorite New Hobby Since Losing 100 lbs
Acting on stage with my boys. I never would have had the confidence to act in front of a crowd when I was overweight. With the weight loss came a new me.

SPIKE LIFE GLOSSARY

Calorie
Compound Exercise
Isolation Exercise
Lactic Acid
Spike Gauntlet
NEAT
TDEE
BMR
BMI
BF%
Law of Thermodynamics
Satiety— the state of being fed, satisfied, or gratified beyond capacity.
Insulin Resistance
Metabolic Syndrome
Essential Amino Acids
Homeostasis
Glucagon
Insulin
Leptin
Glycogen
Crash Diets
Hypoglycemic
Aerobic Threshold

SPIKE DIET X
GLOSSARY

Anabolism – is a metabolic process of consuming energy and building tissue.

BMI – Body Mass Index is formula of height versus weight to determine if you are overweight or obese.

BMR – Basal Metabolic Rate is our resting metabolism. It is our calories expended daily to perform essential bodily functions.

Body-fat percentage – (BF%) is the amount of body-fat we have on our body compared to our overall weight.

Calorie - A calorie is a unit of measurement used to describe the energy in food. A calorie is the amount of energy needed to raise the temperature of one gram of water by one degree Celsius.

Calorie back-loading – is a way of meal planning that allows for the majority of our daily calories to be consumed in the evening.

Catabolism – is a metabolic process of breaking substances down and creating energy.

Compound exercise – This is an exercise that works more than one muscle group. An example is a bench press. It initiates muscle tissues in our chest, shoulders, and triceps.

DOMS – is delayed onset muscle soreness. It's muscle soreness that happens 24-48 hours after you exercise while your body is repairing broken down muscle tissue.

Empty Calories – are calories from food that provide little to no nutritional benefit.

Energy Balance – is a point of homeostasis where we consume and expend an equal amount of energy.

EPOC – is excess post-exercise oxygen consumption. This is fat burning metabolic boost that lasts for hours after exercise.

Essential Amino Acids – These are the amino acids our body cannot produce and we need to get them from the foods we eat.

Ghrelin – is a hormone that makes you feel hungry.

Glucagon - A hormone produced by the pancreas that stimulates an increase in blood sugar levels by converting stored energy to glucose. It has the opposite action of insulin.

Glucose – is the sugar our body burns for energy.

Glycemic Load – is a formula used to determine the impact foods will have on blood sugar levels.

Glycogen – Is a stored form of glucose in our muscles and our liver. Glycogen in our muscles is used to provide energy for our muscles and glycogen in our liver can be converted back to glucose to help regulate blood sugar levels.

Homeostasis - The tendency toward a relatively stable equilibrium maintained by physiological processes. An example is our body lowering metabolism when we consume fewer calories to maintain energy balance.

Hypoglycemia –This is deficiency of glucose in the bloodstream that can cause us to feel light headed, dizzy, and sick.

Insoluble Fiber - keep their shape in water. They promote the movement of foods through your digestive system and provide bulking in foods without adding extra calories.

Insulin - A hormone produced by the pancreas that lowers blood sugar levels by storing excess glucose in cells.

Insulin Resistance - is condition in which a person has a lowered level of response to insulin.

Intermittent Fasting – (IF) is a method of meal planning of alternating long periods of fasting and eating. Many IF meal plans are done by fasting during the day and eating all daily calories in a 3-4 hour window in the evening.

Isolation exercise – This is an exercise that only works one muscle group. An example is a bicep curl as it puts most of the emphasis on solely our biceps.

Lactic acid - is produced in the muscles when glucose is broken down during exercise and strenuous muscular activity.

Law of Thermodynamics – As it pertains to diets, this is the law of calories in versus calories out. If we consume more calories than we expend then we store energy and if we consume less calories than we expend we use burn stored energy.

Leptin – A hormone in our fat cells that helps to regulate hunger and fat storage.

MCT Oil – is a saturated fat very unique to other dietary fats. MCT's consist of shorter (medium-length) chains. This structure accounts for the ability of MCT's to stimulate metabolism and increase body temperature. They are converted by the liver to ketones and are not stored as body-fat.

Metabolic Syndrome - is a combination of medical disorders that increase the risk of developing cardiovascular disease and diabetes

Metabolism – is the chemical processes that take place within our body to sustain life.

NEAT – Non Exercise Activity Thermogenics is the calories expended for everything that is not sleeping, eating, or exercise.

Nutrient Dense – are calories from foods that provide plenty of nutritional needs.

Processed Foods – are foods that have been altered from their natural state to provide stability and increase shelf life.

Resistant Starch - Some resistant starches reduce the glycemic load of foods and also contribute to colon and metabolic system health. Resistant starches also increase lipid metabolism and improve insulin sensitivity.

Satiety – The state of being fed, satisfied, or gratified beyond capacity.

Soluble Fiber - Some soluble fibers lose their shape when mixed in water. They reduce cholesterol absorption and contribute to colon health by increasing intestinal fermentation. This leads to better digestive health.

Spiking – is a philosophy of losing and maintaining weight by greatly increasing caloric intake one day a week. Starvation Mode – is a metabolic adaptation in which our body responds to prolonged periods of restricted caloric consumption.

Supplements – are used to aid a great exercise and diet plan but will not compensate for not exercising or eating poorly.

TDEE – Total Daily Energy Expenditure is our total calories expended daily including NEAT, BMR, eating, and exercise.

TEF – Thermic Effect of Food is the increase in our metabolism to process the calories we consume.

VLCD - Very Low Calorie Diets are extreme diets of 500-800 calories a day sometimes prescribed by doctors to extremely obese patients or promoted by other weight loss plans.

REFERENCES

http://www.jacn.org/content/23/5/373.full

Supplements

http://www.webmd.com/sleep-disorders/tc/melatonin-overview

Exercise
http://www.mayoclinic.com/health/exercise/SM00109

http://www.rice.edu/~jenky/sports/anaerobic.threshold.html

Ainsworth BE, et al. 2011 compendium of physical activities: A
second update of codes and MET values. Medicine & Science in
Sports & Exercise. 2011;43:1575.

http://www.acefitness.org/fitfacts/fitfacts_display.aspx?itemid=19

Anaerobic Threshold

- Law of thermodynamics
http://www.ncbi.nlm.nih.gov/pubmed/7068293
http://www.bodyrecomposition.com/nutrition/excess-protein-and-
fat-storage-qa.html
http://www.livestrong.com/article/480415-fat-vs-glycogen/

- Leptin and Spike Day

Effect of Fasting, refeeding, and dietary fat restriction on plasma
leptin levels.
Weigle DS, Barton D, Connor WE, Steiner RA, Soules MR,
Kuijper JL.

The Role of Leptin in Regulating Neuroendocrine Function in
Humans.
Susan Bluher and Christos Mantzoros

The stimulatory effect of leptin on the neuroenocrine reproductive axis of the monkey. Endocrinology 1998 Nov; 139 (11): 4652-62
Finn PD, Cunningham MJ, Pau KY, Spies HG, Clifton DK, Stiener RA.

Leptin regulates pulsatile luteinizing hormone and growth hormone secretion in the sheep. Endocrinology 200 Nov; 141 (11); 3965-75
Nagatani S, Zeny Y, Keisler DH, Foster DL, Jaff CA.

Evidence that glucose metabolism regulates leptin secretion from cultured rat adipocytes. Endocrinology 1998 Feb; 139 (2): 551-8

Mueller WM, Gregoire Fm, Stanhope Kl, Mobbs CV, Mizuno TM, Warden CH, Stern JS, Havel PJ.

Leptin levels in human and rodent: Measurement of plasma leptin and ob RNA in obese and weight reduced subjects. Nat Med 1995 Nov; 1 (11): 1155-61.
Maffei M, Halaas J, Ravussin E, Pratley RE, Lee GH, Zhang Y, Fei H, Kim S, Lallone R,

- Protein
http://www.rice.edu/~jenky/caryn/protein.html

Earl Mindell's Peak Performance Bible, By Carol Colman, Earl Mindell
http://www.associatedcontent.com/article/371448/understanding_the _thermogenic_effects.html?cat=5
Wolfe RR. Et al. Protein supplements and exercise. Am. J. Clin. Nutr. 72:551s-557s, 2000.

http://www.biology.arizona.edu/biochemistry/problem_sets/aa/aa.htm l

Trumbo P, Schlicker S, Yates AA, Poos M; Food and Nutrition Board of the Institute of Medicine, The National Academies. Dietary reference intakes for energy, carbohydrate, fiber, fat, fatty acids, cholesterol, protein and amino acids. *J Am Diet Assoc.* 2002;102(11):1621-1630.

- Carbohydrates and Glycemic Load

http://www.diabetesnet.com/diabetes_food_diet/glycemic_index.php

- Fatty acids and Coconut oil

Kaunitz H, Dayrit CS. Coconut oil consumption and coronary heart disease. Philippine Journal of Internal Medicine, 1992;30:165-171

http://www.huffingtonpost.com/dr-mercola/coconut-oil-benefits_b_821453.html

http://www.mayoclinic.com/health/trans-fat/CL00032

Kaunitz H, Dayrit CS. Coconut oil consumption and coronary heart disease. Philippine Journal of Internal Medicine, 1992;30:165-171

Prior IA, Davidson F, Salmond CE, Czochanska Z. Cholesterol, coconuts, and diet on Polynesian atolls: a natural experiment: The Pukapuka and Tokelau Island studies, American Journal of Clinical Nutrition, 1981;34:1552-1561

Raymond Peat Newsletter, Coconut Oil, reprinted at www.heall.com. http://www.heall.com/body/healthupdates/food/coconutoil.html An Interview With Dr. Raymond Peat, A Renowned Nutritional Counselor Offers His Thoughts About Thyroid Disease

Baba, N 1982. Enhanced thermogenesis and diminished deposition of fat in response to overfeeding with diet containing medium-chain triglycerides, Am. J. Clin. Nutr., 35:379

(Dr. Mary G. Enig, Ph.D., F.A.C.N. Source: Coconut: In Support of Good Health in the 21st Century

Isaacs CE, Litov RE, Marie P, Thormar H. Addition of lipases to infant formulas produces antiviral and antibacterial activity, Journal of Nutritional Biochemistry, 1992;3:304-308.

Isaacs CE, Schneidman K. Enveloped Viruses in Human and Bovine Milk are Inactivated by Added Fatty Acids(FAs) and Monoglycerides(MGs), FASEB Journal, 1991;5: Abstract 5325, p.A1288.

http://www.umm.edu/altmed/articles/omega-6-000317.htm

Mitsuto Matsumoto, Takeru Kobayashi, Akio Takenakaand Hisao Itabashi. Defaunation Effects of Medium Chain Fatty Acids and Their Derivatives on Goat Rumen Protozoa, The Journal of General Applied Microbiology, Vol. 37, No. 5 (1991) pp.439-445.

St-Onge MP, Jones PJ. Greater rise in fat oxidation with medium-chain triglyceride consumption relative to long-chain triglyceride is associated with lower initial body weight and greater loss of subcutaneous adipose tissue, International Journal of Obesity & Related Metabolic Disorders, 2003 Dec;27(12):1565-71.
http://www.ncbi.nlm.nih.gov/pubmed/12975635

Geliebter, A 1980. Overfeeding with a diet of medium-chain triglycerides impedes accumulation of body fat, Clinical Nutrition, 28:595

Fushiki, T and Matsumoto, K Swimming endurance capacity of mice is increased by consumption of medium-chain triglycerides, Journal of Nutrition, 1995;125:531.http://www.coconut-connections.com/hypothyroidism.htm
Barry Groves, PhD. Second Opinions: Exposing Dietary Misinformation: The Cholesterol Myth, parts 1 and 2

Anandan C, Nurmatov U, Sheikh A. Omega 3 and 6 oils for primary prevention of allergic disease: systematic review and meta-analysis. Allergy. 2009 Jun;64(6):840-8. Epub 2009 Apr 7.

Attar-Bashi NM, Li D, Sinclair AJ. alpha-linolenic acid and the risk of prostate cancer. Lipids. 2004;39(9):929-32.

De Spirt S, Stahl W, Tronnier H, Sies H, Bejot M, Maurette JM, Heinrich U. Intervention with flaxseed and borage oil supplements modulates skin condition in women. Br J Nutr. 2009 Feb;101(3):440-5.

Freeman VL, Meydani M, Hur K, Flanigan RC. Inverse association between prostatic polyunsaturated fatty acid and risk of locally advanced prostate carcinoma. Cancer. 2004;101(12):2744-54.

Geppert J, Demmelmair H, Hornstra G, Koletzko B. Co-supplementation of healthy women with fish oil and evening primrose oil increases plasma docosahexaenoic acid, gamma-linolenic acid and dihomo-gamma-linolenic acid levels without reducing arachidonic acid concentrations. Br J Nutr. 2008 Feb;99(2):360-9.

Harris W. Omega-6 and omega-3 fatty acids: partners in prevention. Curr Opin Clin Nutr Metab Care. 2010; 13(2):125-9.

Kankaanpaa P, Nurmela K, Erkkila A, et al. Polyunsaturated fatty acids in maternal diet, breast milk, and serum lipid fattty acids of infants in relation to atopy. Allergy. 2001;56(7):633-638.

Kast RE. Borage oil reduction of rheumatoid arthritis activity may be mediated by increased cAMP that suppresses tumor necrosis factor-alpha. Int Immunopharmacol. 2001;1(12):2197-2199.

Kenny FS, Pinder SE, Ellis IO et al. Gamma linolenic acid with tamoxifen as primary therapy tn breast cancer. Int J Cancer. 2000;85:643-648.

Kris-Etherton PM, Taylor DS, Yu-Poth S, et al. Polyunsaturated fatty acids in the food chain in the United States. Am J Clin Nutr. 2000;71(1 Suppl):179S-188S.

Kupferer EM, Dormire SL, Becker H. Complementary and alternative medicine use for vasomotor symptoms among women who have discontinued hormone therapy. J Obstet Gynecol Neonatal Nurs. 2009 Jan-Feb;38(1):50-9.

Little C, Parsons T. Herbal therapy for treating rheumatoid arthritis. Cochrane Database Syst Rev. 2001;(1):CD002948.

Manjari V, Das UN. Effect of polyunsaturated fatty acids on dexamethasone-induced gastric mucosal damage. Prostaglandins Leukot Essent Fatty Acids. 2000;62(2):85-96.

Menendez JA, del Mar Barbacid M, Montero S, et al. Effects of gamma-linolenic acid and oleic acid on paclitaxel cytotoxicity in human breast cancer cells. Eur J Cancer. 2001;37:402-413. Macro-nutrients and weight loss

Rakel D. Integrative Medicine. 2nd ed. Philadelphia, PA: Saunders, An Imprint of Elsevier: 2007.

Ramsden C, Gagnon C, Graciosa J, et al. Do omega-6 and trans fatty acids play a role in complex regional pain syndrome? A pilot study. Pain Med. 2010; 11(7):1115-25.

Richardson AJ, Puri BK. The potential role of fatty acids in attention-deficit/hyperactivity disorder. Prostaglandins Leukot Essent Fatty Acids. 2000;63(1/2):79-87.

Schirmer MA, Phinney SD. Gamma-linolenate reduces weight regain in formerly obese humans. J Nutr. 2007 Jun;137(6):1430-5.

Senapati S, Banerjee S, Gangopadhyay DN. Evening primrose oil is effective in atopic dermatitis: a randomized placebo-controlled trial. Indian J Dermatol Venereol Leprol. 2008 Sep-Oct;74(5):447-52.

Srivastava A, Mansel RE, Arvind N, Prasad K, Dhar A, Chabra A. Evidence-based management of Mastalgia: a meta-analysis of randomised trials. Breast. 2007 Oct;16(5):503-12. Epub 2007 May 16.

Surette ME, Stull D, Lindemann J. The impact of a medical food containing gamma-linolenic and eicosapentaenoic acids on asthma management and the quality of life of adult asthma patients. Curr Med Res Opin. 2008 Feb;24(2):559-67.

Weaver KL, Ivester P, Seeds M, Case LD, Arm JP, Chilton FH. Effect of dietary fatty acids on inflammatory gene expression in healthy humans. J Biol Chem. 2009 Jun 5;284(23):15400-7. Epub 2009 Apr 9.

Wakai K, Okamoto K, Tamakoshi A, Lin Y, Nakayama T, Ohno Y. Seasonal allergic rhinoconjunctivitis and fatty acid intake: a cross-sectional study in Japan. Ann Epidemiol. 2001;11(1):59-64.

Fats and Fatty Acids in Human Nutrition. Annals of Nutrition and Metabolism, 2009; 55 (1-3).

Siri-Tarino PW, et al. Meta-analysis of prospective cohort studies evaluating the association of saturated fat with cardiovascular disease Am J Clin Nutr 13 January 2010 [epub ahead of print]

Foster GD, Wyatt HR, Hill JO, et al. Weight and metabolic outcomes after 2 years on a low-carbohydrate versus low-fat diet. A randomized trial. Ann Intern Med 2010; 153:147-157.

Atkins RC. Dr. Atkins' New Diet Revolution. New York: Avon Books, 1998.

http://www.cnn.com/2010/HEALTH/11/08/twinkie.diet.professor/index.html

- Fiber

"Diet, Nutrition and the Prevention of Chronic Diseases", Report of a Joint WHO/FAO Expert consultation, Technical Report Series 916. Dietitians Association of Australia, Smart Eating – Fibre (updated November 2005)
http://www.daa.asn.au/index.asp?PageID=2145834403

http://jn.nutrition.org/content/129/7/1434.full.pdf

- Cravings and hunger

Anderson, G.H., and Woodend, D., "Effect of glycemic carbohydrates on short-term satiety and food intake," Nutr Rev 2003; 61(5): 17-26

Araya, H., et al., "Short-term satiety in preschool children: a comparison between high protein meal and a high complex carbohydrate meal," Int J Food Sci Nutr 2000; 51(2): 119-124

Blundell, J.E., and MacDiarmid, J.I., "Fat as a risk factor for overconsumption: satiation, satiety, and patterns of eating," J Am Diet Assoc 1997 97(7): S63-S69

Bell, E.A., et al., "Sensory-specific satiety is affected more by volume than by energy content of a liquid food," Phys Behav 2003; 78(4): 593-600

Green, S.M., et al., "Effect of fat- and sucrose-containing foods on the size of eating episodes and energy intake in lean males: potential for causing overconsumption," Eur J Clin Nutr 1994; 48(8): 547-555

Guinard, J-X, and Brun, P., "Sensory-specific satiety: comparison of taste and texture effects," Appetite 1998; 31(2): 141-157

Holt, S.H., et al., "A satiety index of common foods," Eur J Clin Nutr 1995 Sep; 49(9): 675-690

Holt, S.A., et al., "The effects of equal-energy portions of different breads on blood glucose levels, feelings of fullness and subsequent food intake," J Am Diet Assoc 2001; 101(7): 767-773

Marmonier, C., et al., "Effects of macronutrient content and energy density of snacks consumed in a satiety state on the onset of the next meal," Appetite 2000; 34(2): 161-168

Pasman, W.J., et al., "Effect of one week of fiber supplementation on hunger and satiety ratings and energy intake," Appetite 29(1): 77-87

Porrini, M., et al., "Effects of physical and chemical characteristics of food on specific and general satiety," Phys Behav 1995; 57(3): 461-468

Porrini, M., et al., "Evaluation of satiety sensations and food intake after different preloads," Appetite 1995; 25(1): 17-30

http://nutritiondata.self.com/topics/fullness-factor

Rigaud, D., et al., "Effects of a moderate dietary fiber supplement on hunger rating, energy input and faecal energy output in young, healthy volunteers. A randomized, double-blind, cross-over trial," Int J Obes 1987; 11(1): 73-78

Rolls, B.J., and Roe, L.S., "Effect of the volume of liquid food infused intragastrically on satiety in women," Phys Behav 2002; 76(4): 623-631

Janet Polivy, Psychological Consequences of Food Restriction, J American Dietetic Association 9666):589-592 June 1996

Koffler M, Kisch ES, Starvation diet and very-low-calorie diets may induce insulin resistance and overt diabetes mellitus. J Diabetes Complications. 1996 Mar-Apr;10(2):109-12.

http://www.thefactsaboutfitness.com/research/leptinmem.htm
Christian Finn, M.Sc. Founder, The Facts About Fitness Ltd.

- Failure & Burn
http://www.annals.org/content/148/10/747.abstract

Summary of studies on Metabolic Adaptation and my Spike Days

Study #1 - (Coleman et al, Diabetologia 42: 636-646, 1999)
- During a 52-96 hour fast, subjects experienced a 4% loss in body mass, accompanied by a 54-72% decline in Leptin concentrations.
- In some subjects, once Leptin declined, the authors administered a glucose infusion (5% solution totaling 338 kcal/day), causing Leptin to increase by 80%, relative to that large depression. This demonstrates that a small <u>carbohydrate</u> load can almost normalize depressed Leptin concentrations.
- It's important to note that this small addition of carbohydrate is only associated with an increase in Leptin concentrations during a fast. During a normal diet phase, I doubt a small carb increase will increase Leptin concentrations.
- In other subjects, after the 4-day fast, only 12 hours of "refeeding" returned Leptin to baseline, demonstrating that acute feeding is an important regulator of Leptin concentrations.

Study #2 - (Kolaczynski et al Diabetes 45: 1511-1515, 1996).
- During the first part of this study, researchers found that after 36h of fasting, Leptin decreased by 77% while after 60h of fasting, Leptin decreased by 82%.
- During the second part of the study (the data plotted above), authors found that Leptin decreased by 20% after 12h and 65% after 36h of fasting. However after 12 h of refeeding, Leptin increased to 62% of normal and after 24h refeeding, leptin increased to 100% of normal.
- This data indicates that 12h fasting is sufficient to reduce serum leptin dramatically - this is concomitant with decreased <u>insulin</u> and increased glucagon, cortisol, catecholamines, and GH. They also indicate that a normal single meal has negligible impact on leptin - it takes prolonged feedings to impact Leptin concentrations.
- Finally, in this study the authors demonstrated that after an overnight fast with a small amount of glucose infusion, Leptin doesn't drop at all.

Study #3 - (Kolaczynski et al J Clin Endocrinol Metab 81 4162-4165, 1996).

- In <u>Part 1</u>, subjects were ridiculously overfed as follows: over 12 hours, subjects ate 120kcal/kg (about 12000kcal for a 100kg individual).
- During the 5th to 10th hour of overfeeding, there was a 40% increase in Leptin that persisted through the morning and continued beyond. Unfortunately, the researchers only measured out Leptin levels until the morning. We don't know how long the Leptin remained elevated. These data indicate that with very big, "Victor Richards type" overfeedings, elevations in Leptin concentrations may persist even after an overnight fast.
- In <u>Part 2</u>, subjects ate 25kcal/kg (2500kcal for a 100kg individual) above normal intake until they gained an additional 10% body mass. During this study, fasting Leptin tripled in response to weight gain (there was a varied response, though: in subjects that gained the most fat, Leptin increased the most).

Study #4 - (Dallongeville et al Int J Obesity 22, 728-733, 1998)
- Leptin increased by 27% over an 8h post meal period while it decreased by 29% during a similar fasted period (these results were obtained during daytime feeding/fasting). These data weren't simply circadian due to the fact that similar changes were seen during nighttime feeding/fasting where Leptin increased by 37% over 8h when fed, and decreased by 27% over 8h when fasting. These data indicate that meal feeding during a normal circadian cycle increases Leptin concentrations while fasting decreases them.

Studies #5 - #7 - (Evans et al Clin Sci London 100(5) 493-498, 2001; Coppack et al Proc Nutr Soc 57 461-470; Dirlewanger et al Int J Obes Relat Metab Disord 11 1413-1418, 2000)
- These studies show that CHO are necessary to induce postprandial Leptin increases, as fat alone doesn't increase Leptin after meals. They also demonstrate that mixed meals are sufficient to induce Leptin increases. Fat doesn't have to be avoided.

BE STRONG & COURAGEOUS

I want to thank you for buying my book. I know how overwhelming wanting to lose weight can be. That's why it's so important to take it one day at a time and forget about being perfect. There's nothing that can stop you from making the same kind of transformation I did.

Remember, our only limitations are our beliefs.

God Bless,

Russell Branjord

HOW TO CONNECT WITH ME

- FACEBOOK.COM/SPIKEDIET
- SPIKEDIET@GMAIL.COM
- SPIKEGUY.COM

About the Author

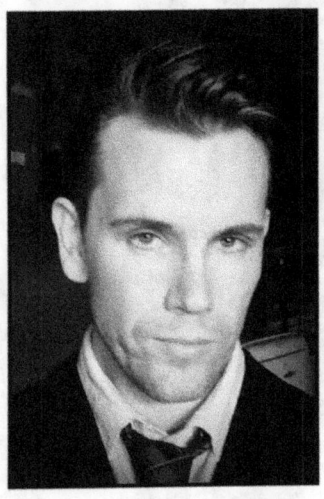

"Spike Guy" **Russell Branjord**, CPT, CFNC, is a published author, certified fitness nutrition coach and an emerging influencer in the weight loss industry.

A living testament of the Spike System, Russ battled obesity for most of his life before experiencing the dietary revelation that led him to create and share the Spike lifestyle.

Russ has been featured on television, radio shows, in newspapers, and has published fitness articles on Thought Catalog and other major health and fitness websites.

Check Russell's availability to speak to your group, online coaching, connect with his social media profiles, and learn more about living the Spike Life at SpikeGuy.com

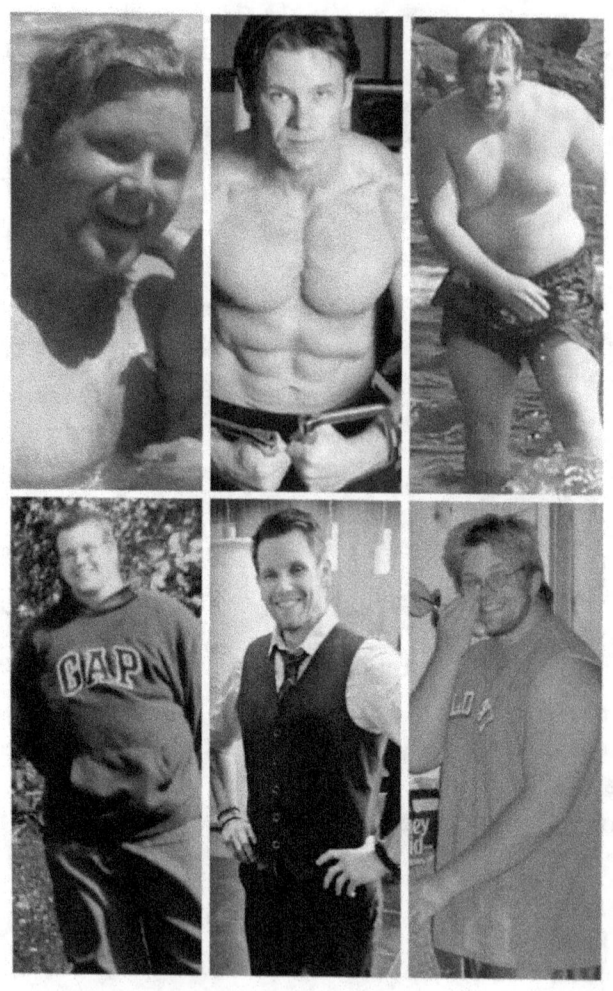

"WITH GOD ALL THINGS ARE POSSIBLE" –
MATTHEW 19:26